the gluten-free revolution

Skyhorse Publishing books may be purchased in bulk at special discounts for sales promotion, corporate gifts, fund-raising, or educational purposes. Special editions can also be created to specifications. For details, contact the Special Sales Department, Skyhorse Publishing, 307 West 36th Street, 11th Floor, New York, NY 10018 or info@skyhorsepublishing.com.

Skyhorse® and Skyhorse Publishing® are registered trademarks of Skyhorse Publishing, Inc.®, a Delaware corporation.

Visit our website at www.skyhorsepublishing.com.

10 9 8 7 6 5 4 3 2 1

Library of Congress Cataloging-in-Publication Data

Shannon-Karasik, Caroline.

The Gluten-Free Revolution: a balanced guide to a gluten-free lifestyle through healthy recipes, green smoothies, yoga, pilates, and easy desserts!/Caroline Shannon-Karasik.

pages cm Includes bibliographical references and index.

ISBN 978-1-62636-275-8 (hardcover: alk. paper)

1. Gluten-free diet—Recipes. 2. Nutrition. 3. Physical fitness.

I. Title. RM237.86.S538 2014 641.3—dc23

2013025663

Cover design by Brian Peterson
All photographs © Caroline Shannon-Karasik

Print ISBN: 978-1-63220-637-4
Ebook ISBN: 978-1-63450-138-5

Printed in China

Caroline Shannon-Karasik

the gluten-free revolution

A Balanced Guide to a Gluten-Free Lifestyle through Healthy Recipes, Green Smoothies, Yoga, Pilates, and Easy Desserts!

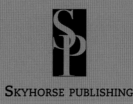

SKYHORSE PUBLISHING

For Mom, who never, ever stopped believing. I am because you are.

table of contents

1   INTRODUCTION

2   What's The Gluten-Free Revolution?
5   My Influence
6   So, What Can I Eat?
7   What Will I Need?
8   Fitness: Scoring the Gluten-Free Bod
10   Join the Revolution

12   CHAPTER ONE: GETTING STARTED

13   Prep Your Kitchen
18   Essential Kitchen Gadgets
19   Fast & Cheap Tools
21   Scoring Deals on Home & Food Items

22   CHAPTER TWO: THE RECIPES

23   Sips & Smoothies
28   Build-Your-Own (BYO) Smoothie
29   Juicing versus Blending

39   Breakfast
53   How to Caramelize an Onion

61   Dressings, Marinades & Toppings
63   How to Pair Greens & Dressings

71   Just a Bite
91   Salads & Sides
103   The Main Event
139   Something Sweet

160   CHAPTER THREE: THE LIFESTYLE

161   Let's Get Physical
163   Take-'Em-Anywhere Yoga Poses
169   4 Yoga Poses for Reducing Head Pain
173   Drool-Worthy Sleepy Time Yoga Sequence
179   On Running
185   15-Minute Cardio Pilates Workout
191   5 Ballet-Inspired Exercises for a Perky Booty
200   Mirror, Mirror
201   Gluten-Free Beauty
202   3 Ways to Use Green Tea for Glowing Skin
204   Make-At-Home Coffee Scrub

206   The Gluten-Free Revolution's Favorites

217   INDEX

225   ACKNOWLEDGMENTS

introduction

welcome to the gluten-free revolution. who's ready to discover balanced, healthful bliss?

What's the Gluten-Free Revolution?
Much like the age-old saying that it's important to "never say never," my way of healthy living stems from the idea that there is not a one-size-fits-all prescription for achieving total wellness. When I launched my blog, *The G-Spot Revolution*, in January 2011, I did so with that theory in mind, creating my mantra "because a healthy life shouldn't be hard to find."

Yeah, it was a bit cheeky—and I meant for it to be that way. But I also wanted to give people the opportunity to define what "G" meant to them: Gorgeous? Grain-free? Gluten-free? Glowing? Green?

The definition was up to the reader.

Prior to my diagnosis with celiac disease in 2010, I spent a large portion of my life subscribing to an all-or-nothing approach. The same characteristics that made me driven and motivated had also often left me unable to relax the rules. There was never room for a happy medium or "sweet spot" in my world. Exercise didn't count unless it was done for at least an hour. If I was trying to minimize sweets, they had to be completely wiped out of the kitchen—not a single granule in sight.

This, of course, led to a constant up-and-down effect throughout my teenage years and early twenties. Unable to maintain the harsh parameters I had set for myself, I would eventually fail at my grand ol' plan, caving to an entire chocolate cake instead of taking the one or two bites I had wanted earlier in the week.

It was a recipe for disaster and I was the main ingredient.

It wasn't until I was able to admit to these patterns that I realized *I* was the root of my inability to maintain a healthy path. *Me! It was all me!* By setting these strict standards, I was like a semitrailer truck careening around a rather curvaceous road—it just wasn't going to end pretty.

I created my philosophy as not only an answer for each one of you, but as a personal lifeline. When I found out that gluten was out and gluten-free was in, I was determined to not let this new restriction rule my life. Sure, I would now have to opt out of Oktoberfest, and cupcakes from my favorite bakery were completely off limits. But I decided right then and there that it was time to subscribe to *a way of life*—not a temporary fix—and I want you to do the same.

I promise, sweet cupcakes, that this is the place where you will find healthful bliss. You are about to uncover the ultimate sweet spot where you can enjoy vibrant green smoothies and have your gluten-free cake too.

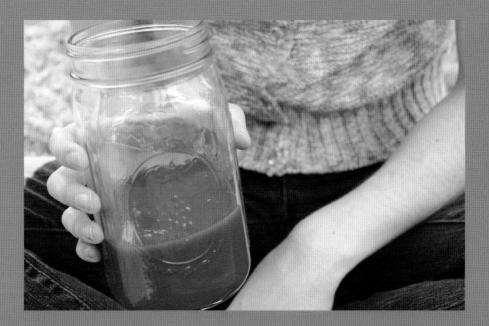

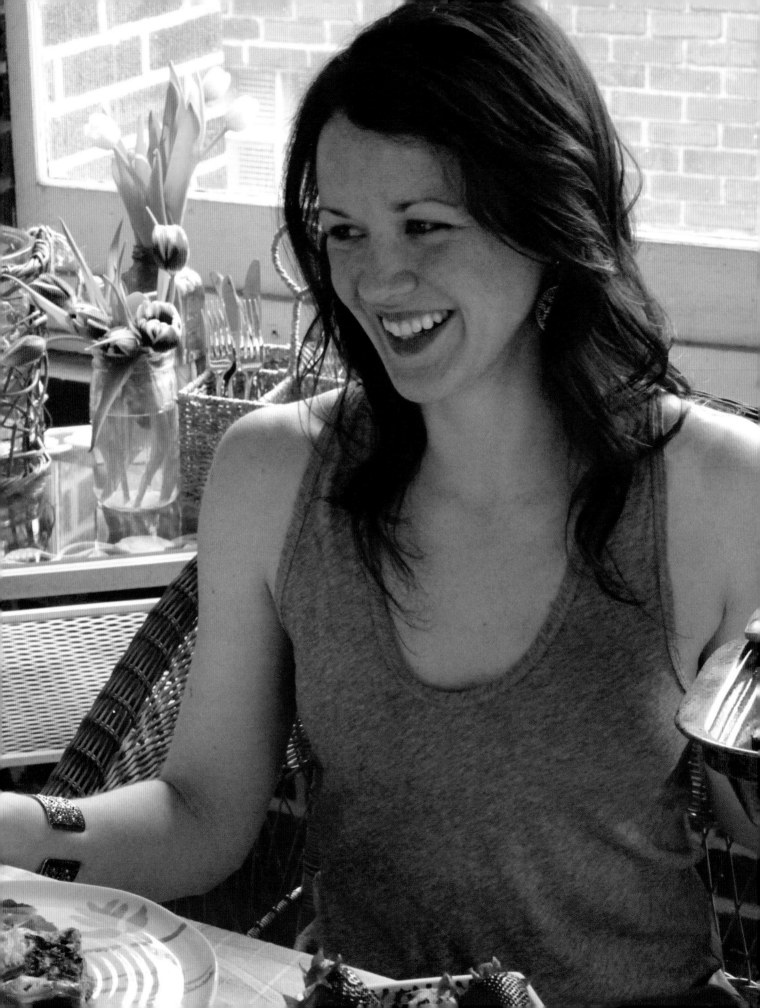

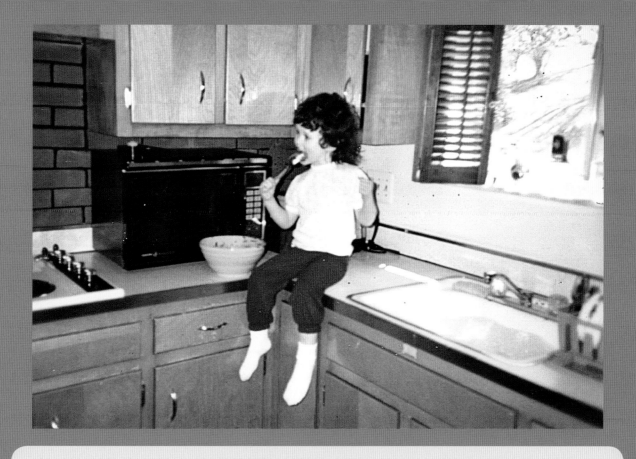

My Influence

As I was growing up, I had no idea that my parents were ahead of the game when it came to health and fitness. Listen, you might think you are obsessed with hummus now, but I was the only kid who showed up to lunch in the third grade with a cucumber, sprouts, and hummus whole grain sandwich.

At the time, I thought my mom was *Oh, my GAWD, so embarrassing* for packing me that lunch. How dare she think I was cool enough to pull off carrots sticking out of my sandwich? The nerve!

But as I grew older, I realized my parents were setting a standard for living that was something I would not only carry with me throughout life, but use to teach other people about just how gorgeous this gluten-free life can be.

My mom was the woman who had chocolate chip brownies mixing in one section of the kitchen and a salad-chopping station happening in the other. Mom was an ardent reader of health books, but she also enjoyed a reasonable dose of fashion and celebrity gossip magazines. She was the embodiment of the lifestyle to which I personally subscribe: healthy, delicious, balanced, and with a touch of something naughty thrown in there, too.

So, if I haven't said it already, then I will say it now: Thanks, Mom and Dad. I would do all of those red-faced elementary lunch days over again to get exactly where I am right now.

So, What Can I Eat?

Let's start with this: The only absolute we will be dealing with in this book is that **everything is gluten-free**. Each recipe includes ingredients that are safe for people with celiac disease or a gluten-intolerance.

Other than that, these recipes are yours for the taking. I often don't do well with words like "never" or "always" and these recipes take into consideration that you might not either. Want to be a vegan? You go girl! There are oh-so-many options for you in this book. Think you'll die without dairy? Don't worry—there are plenty of cheesy options for you.

What you will notice in this book is a bevy of recipes that are based loosely around a high vegan, somewhat Mediterranean diet. I chose to design the book this way because I don't believe in promoting a lifestyle other than the one that I live every day of my life.

My diet revolves around fresh veggies and fruits, gluten-free whole grains, wild fish on occasion, raw nuts, local artisan cheeses, and, naturally, something to quell my very needy sweet tooth.

Does that mean you can't swap certain ingredients for something else? Absolutely not! In fact, you will notice that I provide oodles of tips throughout the book for substitutions that work with each recipe.

If you're curious about some of my favorite products or where you might discover specific brands for ingredients I use in recipes, then you should refer to The Gluten-Free Revolution's Favorites located in the back of this book. Nifty, huh?!

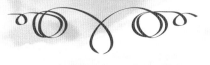

What Will I Need?

When I was putting this book together, another factor that was really important to me was that the recipes didn't require fancy tools or make you feel like a stressed-out Betty. Sure, I adore juicing just as much as the next person, but I know what it's like to be strapped for cash and unable to shell out several hundred dollars for fancy kitchen equipment. That being said, you'll notice that the tools I require are rather basic, leaving the decision to splurge or save up to you.

Check out the pantry essentials and recommended tools sections for stellar items that I like to regularly keep on hand.

Fitness: Scoring the Gluten-Free Bod

Go ahead and say it now, "But I don't have time!"

Listen, I'm going to be frank for a moment: Cut the crap. We both know that booty isn't going to lift and tone itself. That's why I approach gluten-free living as an entire lifestyle and not simply a dietary change.

Now, before you list for me all of the reasons you can't spare a moment to work out, keep in mind that I know you're a busy bee.

I know that when your alarm clock sounds at 5 a.m. for a gym session, the snooze button is suddenly your best friend. I also know what it's like to arrive home to a partner or kiddo who needs your attention. Oh, and I'm very familiar with the *I'll-start-tomorrow* frame of mind.

Truth? You probably won't. You know it and I know it. There's always another reason for why "starting tomorrow" gets pushed to the next day. Promise.

Still, that doesn't mean that a fitness routine has to rule your life. In fact, it can actually be fun if you approach it the right way. I know what you're thinking: *This girl is sippin' too much green juice in da health club . . .*

But, seriously, the right fitness decisions for your life can make all the difference in how you feel about a solid sweat sesh. That's why I am giving you options for working out at home, in the office, at the gym, or on-the-go. I'm not asking for huge time commitments. Just a bit of time to honor your body and show it who's boss (that's you in case you were wondering).

Check out the lifestyle section (see page 160) for tips from yoga, Pilates, and other fitness experts, and learn how you can squeeze in exercise during everyday activities, like watching television or cooking dinner.

"I'm not telling you it is going to be easy—I'm telling you it is going to be worth it."
—anonymous

Join the Revolution

Before we dig into the goodies, I want you to keep a few rules in mind while we journey down this path. I know, I know—I said rules are out and revolting is in. And it so is.

However, these are a few parameters that will set you straight down the path of living a fearlessly healthy and balanced life.

1. **You are now on an un-diet.** Stop counting calories and worrying about the latest fads. If you regularly eat whole, healthy, nutrient-rich foods, then you are making fantastic decisions for your body. 'Nuff said.
2. **Indulge.** Don't get me wrong: I love my greens and whole grains, and they make up a large portion of my diet. But a glass of wine, chocolate, cheesy potatoes, and other naughty items are also a part of my life. Just don't eat them all in one sitting. Unless you are singing the breakup blues. If that's the case, then eat them all. Twice.
3. **Eating healthy doesn't have to be hard.** You've heard it before and you'll hear it again: *"I don't have time for that health food stuff."* Yes, you do. I promise you do. The problem is that no one ever showed you that it doesn't have to be so damn hard. Green smoothie? Minutes. Bodacious salad? No problem. We aren't aiming to be rocket scientists here, so stop making it harder than it has to be.
4. **Focus on your plate.** I love food—period. I can clean a packed plate in no time. But that doesn't mean I should. We live in a world where phones are brought to the dinner table and dining is a recreational activity. While there's certainly room for packing it in like a champ and starting fresh the next day, it's important to more often than not pay attention to the food in front of you. There have been one too many times in my life where I have shoveled something in so that I can quickly move on to the next thing. Not good, people. Take it slow and savor your food as much as you can.

5. **Stop with the drama.** Nix as much negative energy as you can from your life and you will recover more than just your sanity. The fact is, your diet and energy also suffer when you are dealing with stress. Yes, difficult situations will crop up now and then. But that friend who is constantly complaining to you about work, her husband, the crossing guard who looked at her funny? Believe it or not, she's bringing you down too. Make a commitment to get healthy together or swap long conversations with her for a walk outside. Your body will thank you.

The truth is, more often than not we are either being too hard or too easy on ourselves. Some of us are a Strict Sally in the kitchen, leaving no room for food fun, while others routinely subscribe to the *I'll start tomorrow* philosophy. Neither one of these lifestyles will work in the long haul because they are sitting on extreme ends of the well-being spectrum.

Whether you need to be reassured that it's OK to have a piece of chocolate after dinner, or you're the chica who seriously needs a kick in the pants, we're about to help you get there. Ready to join the revolution? Let's rock 'n' roll, sweet pea.

Chapter One:
Getting Started

Prep Your Kitchen

I am a firm believer in the idea that food preparation doesn't have to require a culinary degree. With a little bit of finesse and the right ingredients, you can easily have a healthy dinner on the table or become the next gluten-free baking goddess on the block.

This is a list of my favorite items to keep in my pantry, refrigerator, and freezer. Many of them are things you will already have on hand, while a few are ingredients that you will acquire along the way. Don't go out and buy them all at once. Instead, budget your dough and purchase certain things as you need them for a recipe or when you simply want to try something new.

Important: All of these items listed should also be gluten-free if you are adhering to a strict gluten-free diet. Check with individual manufacturers for any questions about ingredients. If you have other intolerances, allergies, or special dietary needs, then you should also do your homework.

For specific gluten-free brands I love, see The Gluten-Free Revolution's Favorites in the back of this book.

PANTRY
Herbs and Seasonings
- Sea salt
- Pepper
- Cumin
- Garam masala
- Chili powder
- Red pepper flakes
- Paprika
- Rosemary

- Thyme
- Oregano
- Ground cinnamon
- Nutmeg
- Garlic Powder

Oils and Vinegars
- Olive oil
- Toasted sesame oil
- Grapeseed oil
- Apple cider, red, white, and/or balsamic vinegar
- Tamari or soy sauce

Grains and Pasta
- **Quinoa:** Red, white, or rainbow, it's a power grain that is useful in a number of baking and side dish recipes.
- **Rice:** Brown, jasmine, basmati, and arborio
- **Quinoa or brown rice pastas:** My go-to dish on busy nights.

Baking Essentials
- **Gluten-free flours:** I regularly use almond meal, brown and white rice flour, tapioca flour, cornstarch, and arrowroot starch.
- **Maple syrup:** A favorite for gluten-free pancakes and also an ingredient I use often in my baking recipes.
- **Pumpkin puree:** Make sure it's pure pumpkin (no added ingredients).
- **Unsweetened, natural applesauce:** Another baking "must" in my house.
- **Chocolate chips:** Choose a gluten-free and/or vegan brand.
- **Sugar:** Granulated, brown, and coconut sugars are all good to have on hand for various baked goods.
- **Handy add-ins:** Non-stick cooking spray, baking powder, baking soda, pure coco powder, pure honey, pure vanilla extract, and unsweetened, shredded coconut

Handy Extras

- **Plant-based protein powder and raw cacao powder:** Two of my favorite smoothie add-ins.
- **Raw nuts:** I typically have a range of raw nuts on hand, including walnuts, almonds, pistachios, pecans, pignolias, and cashews.
- **Vegetable broth:** Swap water for vegetable broth when boiling rice or quinoa for a bit of flavor.
- **Natural nut butters:** Almond, peanut, and cashew are a few of my favorites. Sunflower seed butter is a great option for people who are allergic to peanuts or tree nuts.
- **Pesto:** It's fun and easy to make your own, but sometimes the food processor feels like a hassle. When that's the case, grab for this and toss it with your favorite gluten-free pasta.
- **Gluten-free oats:** I am obsessed with granola, and if you are too, then you might want to have these on hand.
- **Canned beans:** Chickpeas, black beans, black-eyed peas, red kidney beans, and butter beans are all good options.
- **Canned diced tomatoes and pasta sauce:** Use for pasta dishes or other recipes, like chili.

REFRIGERATOR

Vegetables

- **Avocados:** One of my favorite additions to salads, rice bowls, and smoothies.
- **Potatoes** (sweet, red, purple, yellow, etc.): Roasted, mashed, stuffed—potatoes are delish.
- **Garlic:** I regularly use garlic in recipes—it's one of my favorite additions to a dish.
- **Parsley:** Throw it in smoothies or on top of a dish for a fresh kick.
- **Yellow, Red, and Green Onions:** Just have 'em.
- **Fresh Vegetables:** Carrots, celery, broccoli, asparagus, Brussels sprouts, and whatever else you might like. Have two or three of them on hand, giving

you no excuse to leave veggies out of a dish. Fresh cut vegetables are also a great option for a healthy snack.

- **Spinach:** Use it for smoothies, salads, or as a dinner side dish. In one week, I go through more spinach than I care to admit.
- **Other greens:** I'm talking lettuces, arugula, kale, and mustard, dandelion and collard greens. Have two or three of them on hand for various recipes.

Fruits

- **Apples:** Eat 'em with peanut butter, a bit of cheese, or solo for a solid snack.
- **Bananas:** Keep them on the counter until they are ripe for eating. Too ripe? Freeze them for future baking projects.
- **Cherry tomatoes:** You can, of course, choose whatever tomatoes you like, but I think these are the most useful for a variety of recipes.
- **Lemons & Limes:** Add a great pop of flavor to a variety of dishes.
- **Other fruits:** Berries, grapes, grapefruit, nectarines, and other fruits are good to have on hand when they are in season.

Other Items

- **Eggs:** If you are going to eat 'em, then try to get as down-to-earth as possible. I'm talking free-range, locally farmed eggs. The more you know who is farming your eggs, the better.
- **Dairy-free milk:** Almond, coconut, hemp, flaxseed, etc.
- **Natural or dairy-free cheeses:** I love to have cheddar, goat, and feta cheeses on hand. Try to buy local brands if they are available at your supermarket. If you are a vegan or simply can't tolerate lactose, then choose a tasty dairy-free brand.
- **Spirulina powder:** Smoothie addition! See page 28.
- **Flaxseed meal:** Add to smoothies and use for baking.
- **Mustard:** Whole grain, honey, and Dijon mustards are all useful in various recipes.

- **Fresh herbs:** Basil, thyme, oregano, and sage are a few of my favorite fresh herbs.
- **Red curry paste:** Spice things up with a bit of Thai flavor.
- **Yogurt:** Greek, soy, coconut, or good old-fashioned, yogurt is not only a yummy breakfast choice, but it also doubles as a helpful baking ingredient.
- **Hummus:** Choose your favorite gluten-free brand and have it on hand for quick snacking.
- **Ketchup:** I'm from Pittsburgh—did you really think I could leave that one out? Do me a favor, however, and think of this condiment as a treat. It packs a high sugar content.
- **Mayo:** Regular, light, vegan—choose a spread that makes you smile.
- **Salad dressing:** Have one or two on hand that might also work double duty as a marinade, like a balsamic vinaigrette.
- **Extra firm tofu:** Use it in a number of vegetarian and vegan recipes.
- **Smoothie add-ins:** Udo's oil, coconut oil, and hemp seed (see page 23 for ideas)

FREEZER

- **Frozen vegetables:** Corn, edamame, peas, green beans, cauliflower, okra, and broccoli are just a few of the frozen veggies I have in my freezer at any given time. Not only are they helpful in recipes like soups and chili, but they are also a fantastic option when I'm pressed for time.
- **Frozen fruit:** In my opinion, this is a key ingredient for creamy and delicious smoothies. Choose strawberries, peaches, pineapple, or whatever other fruit you are craving.
- **Veggie burgers:** A lunchtime essential in my house, especially when I'm out of leftovers and lengthy food prep isn't an option.
- **Wild fish:** I don't rely on it as a regular, but when I am craving fish, I like to have some in the freezer that I can quickly thaw and pop on the grill.
- **Gluten-free bread:** I love a good sandwich every now and then. Keeping my gluten-free bread in the freezer helps it to last longer. That way, I only take out what I need and the rest stays frozen.

Essential Kitchen Gadgets

This is the section where I tell you all of the expensive gadgets you have to buy in order to make your kitchen complete. *Kidding!* Just like my belief that food preparation doesn't have to be a time-intensive project, I also think kitchen tools can be pared down to include a few necessities that make cooking and baking fun. Do we all love to have some fun in the kitchen section every now and then? Sure. That's why I included a few "splurge" recommendations in case you choose to cash your paycheck for a fancy blender.

But all of the recipes in this book can be made with the tools that are listed in the "save" category, meaning you will not only have fun in the kitchen, but you will also still have money left to eat. Go you!

Fast & Cheap Tools

These tools are essential to every kitchen and are simple to add to your collection. I have even scored some of these in the dollar section at Target. *The prices in parentheses reflect the average cost of each item.*

- Silicone brush ($6)
- Rubber spatula ($5)
- Large mixing spoons ($4–5)
- Wire baking rack ($10)
- Muffin and cupcake pan ($9)
- Set of food prep bowls ($10)
- Baking pan ($11–13)
- Cutting boards ($5–6)
- Set of mixing bowls ($20)
- Peeler ($7–8)

Other Essential Kitchen Items

Blender
Splurge: Vitamix 5200 ($450)
Save: NutriBullet by MagicBullet ($89)

Food Processor
Splurge: KitchenAid 9-Cup Food Processor ($149.99)
Save: Hamilton Beach 10-Cup Food Processor ($50)

Mixer
Splurge: KitchenAid Artisan Series 5-Quart Standing Mixer ($350)
Save: KitchenAid 5-Speed Hand Mixer ($40–45)

Cookware Set
Splurge: Calphalon Contemporary Stainless-Steel 13-Piece Set ($550)
Save: Farberware Reliance 15-piece Set ($60)

Set of Knives
Splurge: Wüsthof Classic 7-Piece Knife Block Set ($300)
Save: J.A. Henckels International Fine Edge Synergy 3-Piece Knife Set ($19.99)

Vegetable "Pasta" Maker
Splurge: Paderno World Cuisine Spiralizer ($36)
Save: OXO Julienne Peeler ($9.99)

Parchment Paper/Baking Mats*
Splurge: Silpat Baking Mat ($25)
Save: Parchment paper ($5)

*Keep in mind: While the initial investment in a baking mat might be pricier than parchment paper, the mat will last for much longer than parchment paper, which is disposed of at the end of each use. If you have a bit of extra cash, then spring for the baking mat—it will last you for a few years, depending on how often you use it.

Scoring Deals on Home & Food Items

My husband, Dan, regularly teases me for the thrill I get from scooping up deals on home decor, health items, and other goods I use on a regular basis. But I am all about a bargain, and it's my theory that a little bit of digging can often turn up a wealth of savings. Here are a few places where I like to check for home, kitchen, and grocery steals.

Department Stores

- **Marshalls, T.J. Maxx, and HomeGoods:** Call me nerdy, but some of my all-time-favorite leisurely Saturdays include trips to these stores to score deals on home goods, such as bowls, placemats, glassware, linens, and utensils.
- **Macy's and Kohl's:** Two great department stores that host fantastic sales on home goods, such as blenders, cookware, and dinnerware. For example, I scored my NutriBullet for $92.99 at Kohls.com after applying a coupon to the already marked down price of $99.99.

Online

- **Vitacost.com:** Score a bevy of deals on supplements, protein powders, beauty products, and more. When I'm looking to try a new health product, this is one of the first places I check. *vitacost.com*
- **Abe's Market:** This online natural market regularly hosts sales on bath and body products, gluten-free goods, and even pet care items. *abesmarket.com*
- **Soap.com & Vine.com:** These sites are just two of a number of online shopping sites within a family of online brands that host deals on healthy beauty products, eco-friendly cleaning products, gluten-free snacks, and baby gear. *soap.com* and *vine.com*

Chapter Two:
The Recipes

This is maybe the best part of the whole book, right? Here's where you will discover a wide range of gluten-free recipes that are designed to fill your health needs and naughty cravings all in a few bites.

Take note that I'm not going to tell you to choose gluten-free ingredients in every single item listed throughout the recipes. To avoid cluttering their natural beauty, it's safe for you to assume that if I mention it, then there's a gluten-free option out there somewhere. Check with individual manufacturers' policies to understand their gluten-free standards and, of course, refer to The Gluten-Free Revolution's Favorites in the back of this book for a list of some of my favorite products.

Ready to dig in? Here we go.

sips & smoothies

Green Machine Smoothie
Strawberry Maca Mint Smoothie
Orange Carrot Ginger Sunrise Smoothie
Raspberry Coffee Pick-Me-Up
Infused Water
Post-Workout Smoothie
Hair & Skin Kiwi Avocado Booster
Beet-iful Ginger Apple Smoothie

One of my favorite ways to start the day is with a green smoothie or plant-based juice. It's my belief that there's no better way to break the sleeping fast (get it? break-fast) than with a dose of vitamin-packed nutrients. Plus, smoothies and other healthy sips can make for a wonderful midday treat.

Green Machine Smoothie (vegan)

Makes 24 ounces

This smoothie is packed with iron-rich spinach, but don't expect to notice—
the fruit masks the "green" taste that might otherwise be a little bitter for
most palates. Top it off with a dose of Udo's Oil (or another plant-based
essential fatty acids oil) for a boost from omega-3 and -6 fatty acids.

ingredients
2–3 handfuls of spinach
1 cup dairy-free milk
1 scoop vegan protein powder
1 cup frozen mixed berries
½ medium banana
½ Tablespoon Udo's Oil (optional)

directions
Put all ingredients into a high-speed blender and mix until thoroughly
combined. Serve immediately.

Strawberry Maca Mint Smoothie (vegan option)
Makes 1 serving

Need an afternoon pick-me-up? While coffee might be your beverage of choice, research shows maca has amazing energizing benefits that just might help work you out of a funk. The superfood is grown in the Andes Mountains of Peru and is a fantastic vegetarian source of B-12. Bonus? The maca's hormone-regulating powers have also been shown to quell PMS symptoms and add a little extra "oomph" between the sheets.

ingredients
1 Tablespoon maca powder
1 Tablespoon honey or maple syrup
5 fresh mint leaves
1 cup frozen strawberries
½ cup unsweetened vanilla dairy-free milk (almond, coconut, hemp, etc.)

directions
Blend all ingredients in a high-speed blender until smooth and serve.

Orange Carrot Ginger Sunrise Smoothie (vegan)
Makes 2 servings

When I was younger, my dad always said, "Eat your carrots—they put hair on your chest!" Every time he said it, I would wrinkle my nose, but he was quick to remind me that carrots were also beneficial to my eye and skin health. Dad knew what he was talking about: Not only do carrots boast those benefits, but they are also rich in calcium and beta-carotene, which are ideal for boosting the immune system and fighting cancer. Pair the root veggies with vitamin C-rich oranges, spicy ginger, and a few other ingredients for this delightfully bright smoothie.

ingredients
1 cup carrots, peeled and cut into ½-inch chunks
2 medium oranges, peeled
½ to 1-inch fresh ginger root, peeled
1 cup frozen mango chunks or peach slices
1 lemon, peeled
1½ cups pure coconut water

directions
Add all ingredients to a high-speed blender and blend until smooth. Serve and enjoy!

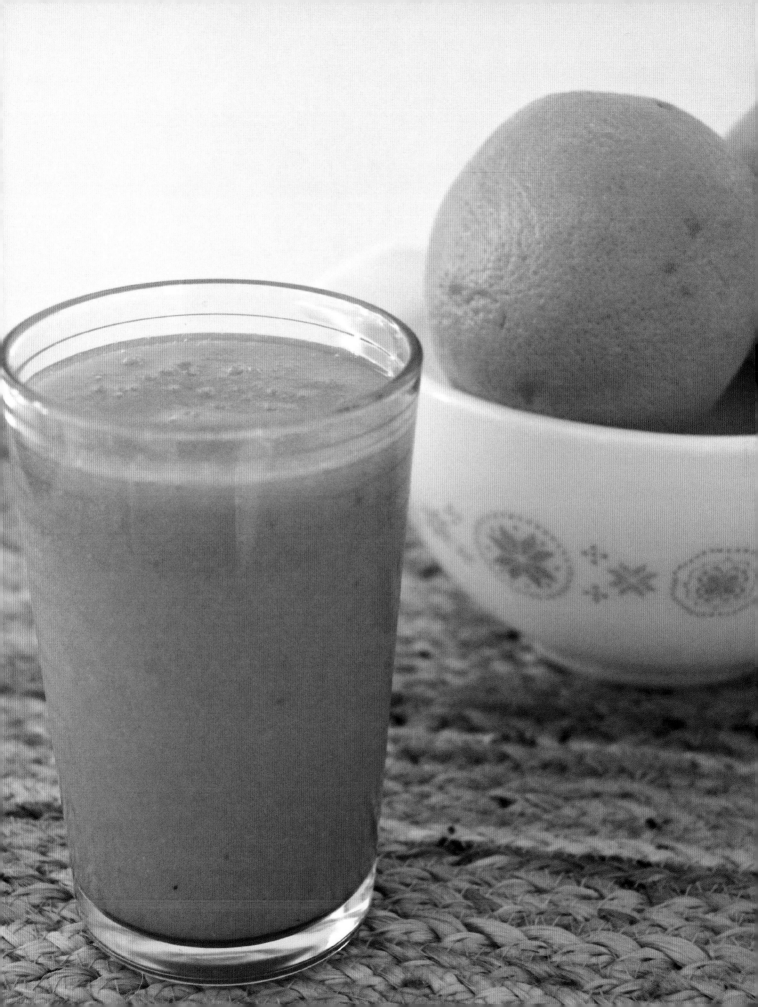

Build-Your-Own (BYO) Smoothie

1. **Get some greens in there.** Leafy green vegetables are a nutrient-packed addition to any smoothie and barely detectable once you add in all of the other ingredients. Choose from 1–2 cups of raw spinach, dandelion and mustard greens, or baby kale. If you are choosing kale, then make sure you get the baby kind because the large leaves can make a smoothie taste like sludge.
2. **Choose a liquid.** This is where I add 1 cup of a dairy-free beverage, like almond, coconut, hemp or flaxseed milk, or even some pure coconut water. Of course, fresh-pressed juice is also an option. If you've blended your smoothie for a bit and it still looks too thick, just add a bit more liquid to it.
3. **Get some fat in there.** I'm talking the healthy kind, like nut butters (peanut, almond, sunflower, or cashew) or flaxseed meal, which is also packed with omega-3s and fiber. Avocado is also a delicious option, giving smoothies a rich and creamy texture. No matter what you choose, add about 2 Tablespoons.
4. **Throw in some fresh or frozen fruit.** This is where you add a bit of sweetness to your smoothie. Bananas, strawberries, raspberries, blueberries, and peaches are all yummy choices. Choose frozen and create a thicker smoothie texture.
5. **Extras! Extras!** I also love to add a smidge of something extra to all of my smoothies. Try chia seeds, cacao powder, spirulina, fresh spearmint or peppermint leaves, or plant-based protein powder to give smoothies a boost.

Did you know? Adding a bit of essential fat to a smoothie can help with the maintenance of necessary nutrients and minerals. That's because fat-soluble vitamins—like vitamin A (sweet potatoes, dried apricots), vitamin K (leafy greens, Brussels sprouts), vitamin E (broccoli and red bell peppers), and vitamin D (fresh fish)—are more easily absorbed and beneficial when mixed with a bit of healthy fat, like flaxseed meal or almonds.

Juicing versus Blending

I absolutely adore juicing, but let's be honest—it's not exactly time efficient. I have a juicer and I use it when I have time, but I opt for smoothies on a more regular basis in an effort to get liquid nutrients on the fly.

juicing

When it comes to using a juicer, the purpose of removing the pulpy fiber from the vegetables and fruits is to send all of those vitamins directly to our bloodstream without having to make the digestion system work (i.e., if there is no fiber to digest, then the body simply has the job of absorbing nutrients).

This is also beneficial when you consider how many fruits and vegetables you would have to eat or blend in order to achieve the concentration of vitamins that are in one serving of juice that comes from a juicer. If the average 32 ounces of juice has 2 cucumbers, 2 broccoli stems, 4 stalks of celery, 1 romaine lettuce heart, 6 kale stalks, an apple, a pear, and more, then imagine trying to squeeze that into a veggie and fruit smoothie—start drinking now because that will take all day! (And your digestive system might just get a little, shall we say . . . antsy?)

Try: Breville Juice Fountain Plus

blending

Blending fruits and veggies has its benefits too. Mushing all of those ingredients into one blended smoothie of healthful activity is incredibly good for your body. However, it will contain fiber and, while that is not a bad thing at all, it will cause your digestive system to get to work.

One very specific benefit of blended fruits and veggies? It's a quick and simple process! Juicing is wonderful but can be time consuming. Blended smoothies are ideal for the guy or gal on the go, and are a great option for squeezing in a healthy nosh on busy mornings.

The fiber in smoothies will also help to slow down blood sugar spikes or the "rush" that can be experienced from drinking straight up juice. This is a factor that is especially beneficial to someone who suffers from diabetes or any other blood sugar imbalance.

Try: Vitamix 5200 Super or NutriBullet

Raspberry Coffee Pick-Me-Up (vegan option)

Makes 1 serving

I love coffee, but I do try to make it a ritual I enjoy as opposed to a habitual activity I require. Still, the truth is some days require an extra jolt. That's where this smoothie comes in. Rich with cacao and a splash of raspberries, this smoothie will appear rather naughty to the untrained eye.

ingredients

1 cup frozen raspberries
¼ cup dairy-free milk (coconut, almond, hemp, flax, etc.)
½ cup cold brewed coffee
2 Tablespoons raw cacao powder
2 Tablespoons honey or agave syrup
shaved dark chocolate (optional)

directions

Blend all ingredients in a high-speed blender and serve cold. Pour into a glass and top with dark chocolate shavings, if desired.

Did you know? The superfood benefits of raw cacao powder include a dosage of antioxidants that is 14 times the amount of those found in red wine!

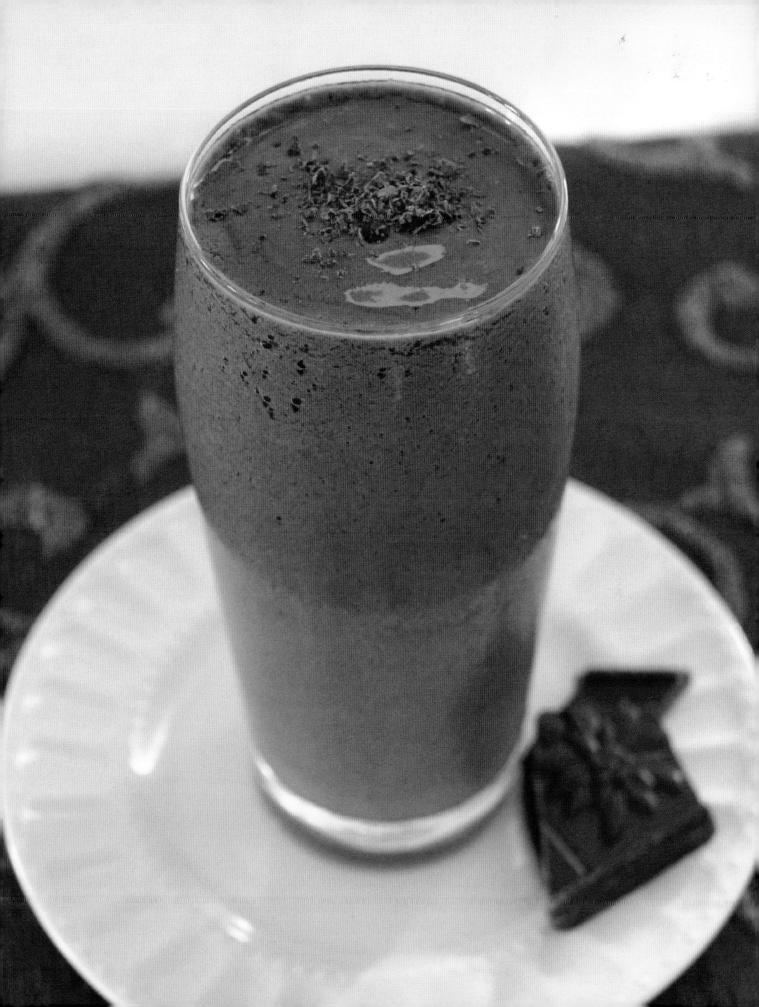

Infused Water

Not only is fruit- and herb-infused water visually stunning, it's also a beautiful idea for getting a springtime party kicked off in style. Choose one or all of these mixes, serving in mason jars for a down-home feel.

Cucumber + Lime

Add a few slices of fresh cucumber and lime to water for a fresh beverage.

Edible Flowers + Orange Slices

Who knew a drink could be so beautiful? Discover edible flowers in your grocery store's produce section and mix them with a few orange slices for a cheerful brew.

Raspberries + Mint

Stir a cup of frozen raspberries into sparkling water, adding fresh mint leaves throughout.

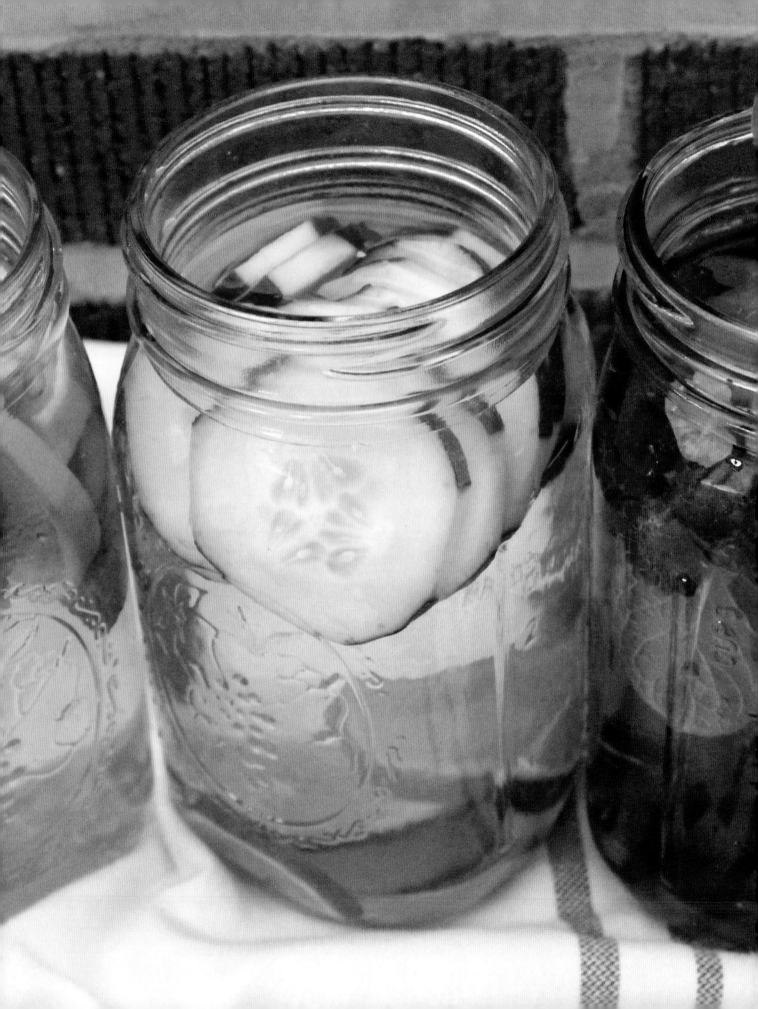

Post-Workout Smoothie (vegan)

Makes 1 serving

I have always envied ladies and dudes who leave the gym looking almost as primped and polished as they did when they first arrived.

Anyone who knows me will tell you that it is absolutely impossible for me to end a workout and look like anything other than a hot mess. My naturally curly hair will be wacky and matted to one side of my head. My face will be flush with a pinkish glow. And I will without a doubt be sweating like a pig (not the cute kind).

Of course, I don't worry about it too much, but I do know that if my appearance is any indication of how hard I have been working, then I'd better be sure to do some post-workout refueling.

This smoothie is one of my favorites, packed with vitamin C, calcium, and coconut water, which gives you an awesome dose of potassium, helping to restore necessary electrolytes that are lost during a sweat session.

ingredients

1 medium orange, peeled
2 cups frozen peaches
1 scoop plant-based vanilla protein powder
16 ounces pure coconut water

directions

Blend all ingredients in a high-speed blender and serve cold.

Hair & Skin Kiwi Avocado Booster

Makes 1 serving

Rich in vitamins C and E, the kiwi fruit is known for its ability to add oomph to lifeless hair and dull skin. Mix it into this smoothie for a refreshing mix that helps build collagen and boost your immune system. The avocado provides a smooth taste and healthy dose of skin-enhancing vitamin E.

ingredients

1 kiwi fruit, peeled
1 lemon, peeled
½ a Bartlett, Bosc, or Anjou pear
5–6 leaves from dandelion greens
1½ cups pure coconut water
½ avocado, peeled and pitted

directions

Blend all ingredients in a high-speed blender and serve cold.

Beet-iful Ginger Apple Smoothie with Strawberries
Makes 2 servings

Beets are superstars when it comes to fortifying blood and boosting our bodies' iron stores. The root veggie is packed with beta-carotene (a major immune booster) and other vitamins and minerals, including folic acid (necessary for the healthy production of red blood cells) and manganese (essential for building bones).

ingredients
1 medium beet (including leaves), scrubbed and cut into quarters
1 organic apple, washed and cut into quarters
1 lemon, peeled
½ to 1-inch fresh ginger root, peeled
1½ cups unsweetened dairy-free milk (almond, coconut, hemp, etc.)
1 cup frozen strawberries

directions
Add all ingredients to a high-speed blender and blend until smooth. Serve and enjoy!

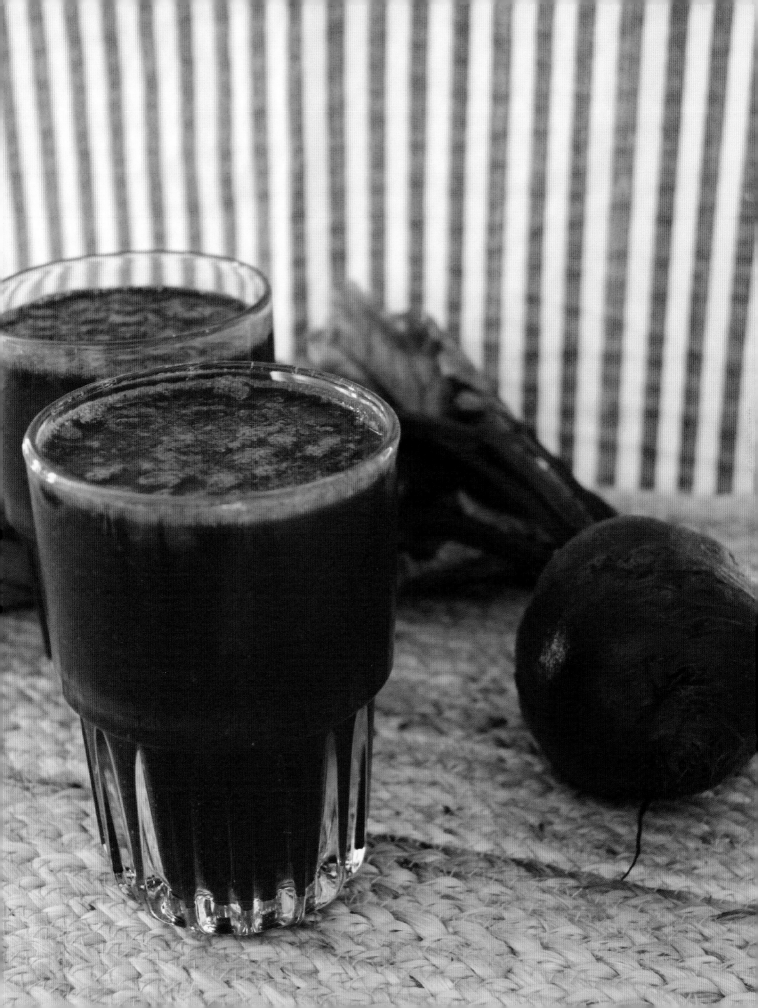

breakfast

Orange Fig Pecan Granola
Tropical Pineapple Yogurt
Peanut Butter Coconut Quinoa Granola
Banana Bread Quinoa Cereal
Raw Sour Cherry Almond Bar
Goat Cheese & Asparagus Quiche Cups
Sweet Potato Spinach Quiche
Mushroom Potato Crust Quiche
Raspberry Lemonade Doughnuts

Morning meals are quite often my favorite dish of the day. I am a firm believer that what I choose to eat for breakfast determines not only the food decisions that will follow, but how I will feel for the rest of the day. It's a sure bet that when I skip breakfast I will turn into a cranky pants and inevitably make a split-second decision when I am able to get my hands on some food. So what if it's a 600-calorie gluten-free brownie? I'm hungry! See the problem? When we're ravenous, logic eventually gives way to *get something in my stomach now!* This, of course, can lead to a series of not-so-healthy food decisions. The moral of this story: Eat your breakfast, people!

Orange Fig Pecan Granola (vegan)

Makes 8½ cups

ingredients
¼ cup maple syrup
½ cup unsweetened, all-natural applesauce
3 cups certified gluten-free oats
¾ cup pecans, chopped
⅓ cup figs, chopped (remove stems if still intact)
¼ cup flaxseed meal
¼ teaspoon sea salt
½ teaspoon vanilla extract
½ teaspoon ground cinnamon
zest of one medium orange

directions
Preheat oven to 300°F. Prepare a baking sheet by lining with parchment paper or baking mat. Place the applesauce and maple syrup in a small pot and warm over medium heat, stirring consistently. Remove from heat and set aside.

In a medium bowl, combine the oats, pecans, figs, flaxseed meal, sea salt, vanilla extract, cinnamon, and orange zest. Pour the applesauce and maple syrup mixture on top of dry ingredients, and stir until ingredients are combined.

Spread the mixture onto the baking sheet and then bake in oven for 55–60 minutes, until golden brown. Toss the granola with a spatula halfway through the bake time.

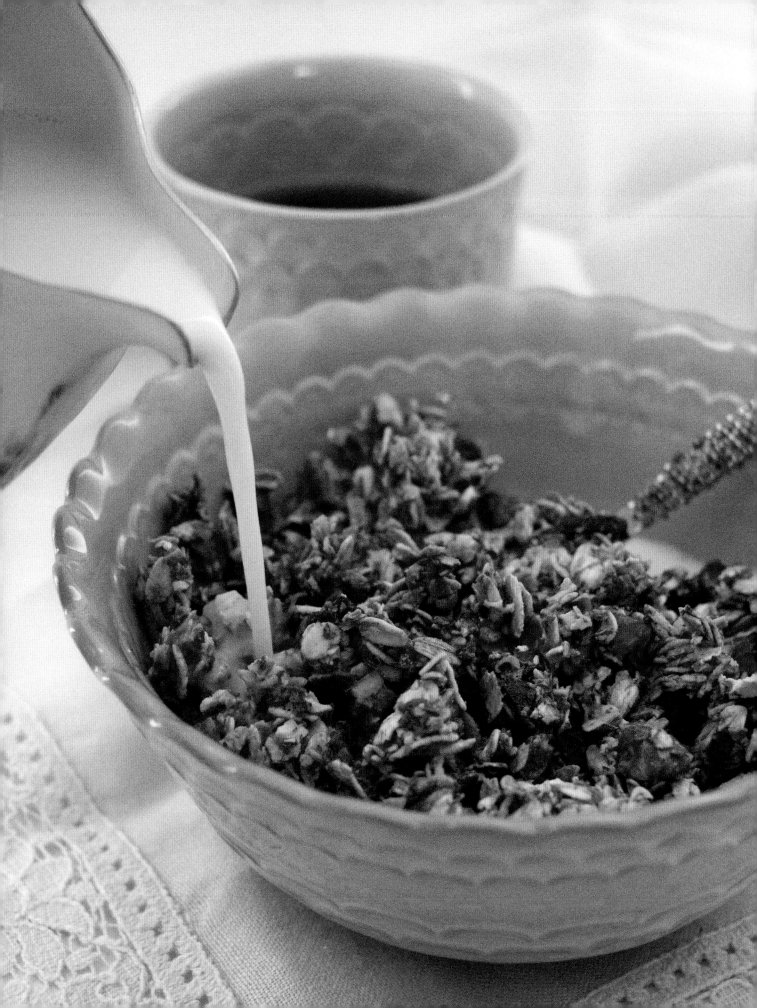

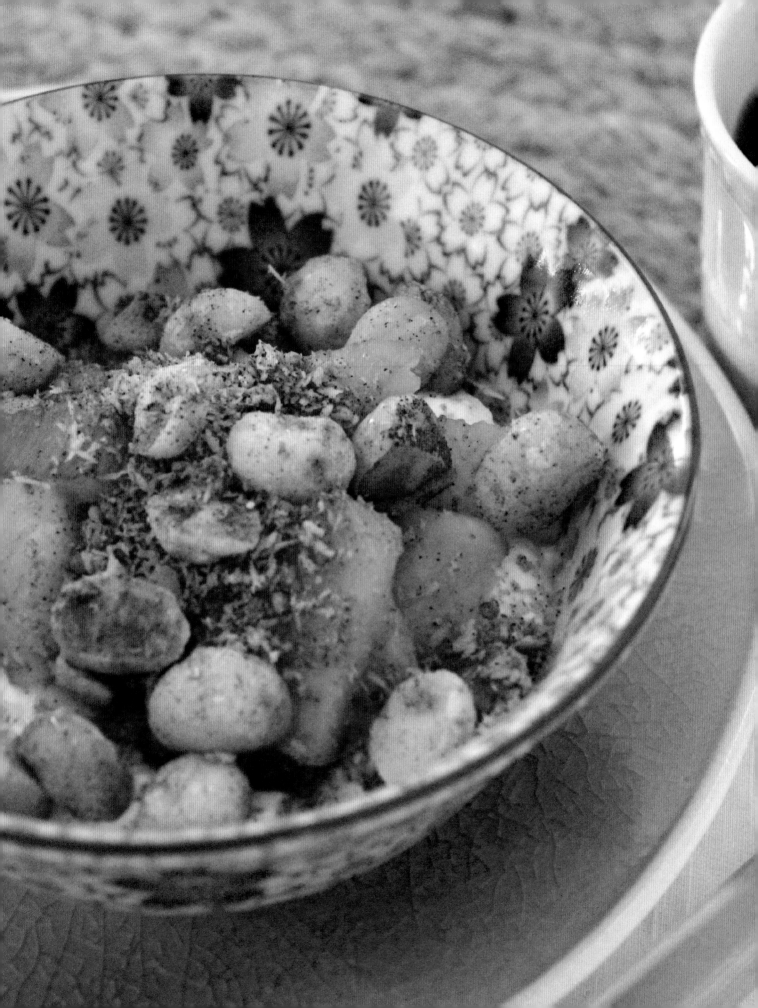

Tropical Pineapple Yogurt with Toasted Macadamia Nuts & Coconut (vegan option)

Makes 1 serving

When Dan and I first visited Sin City, we stayed at the Wynn Las Vegas. Our first morning there was spent at the Terrace Pointe Café, basking in the warm sunshine and drinking bottomless mimosas. Oh, and I also had a delish yogurt that was a lot like this recipe. Absolute heaven in a bowl.

ingredients

6 ounces Greek or vegan yogurt
3 Tablespoons roughly chopped macadamia nuts
2 Tablespoons unsweetened, shredded coconut
¼ teaspoon ground cinnamon
½ cup pineapple, cubed
1 teaspoon coconut oil
drizzled honey (optional)

directions

Preheat oven to 300°F. Scoop yogurt into a bowl and set aside.

In a medium bowl, mix macadamia nuts, coconut, and cinnamon together, then scoop onto a small baking sheet. Toast for 5–7 minutes, or until golden brown. Remove from oven and set aside.

Heat coconut oil in a medium sauté pan over low-medium heat. Add pineapple and sauté for 4–5 minutes, stirring occasionally. Remove from heat.

Top yogurt with pineapple, macadamia nut mixture, and honey, if desired.

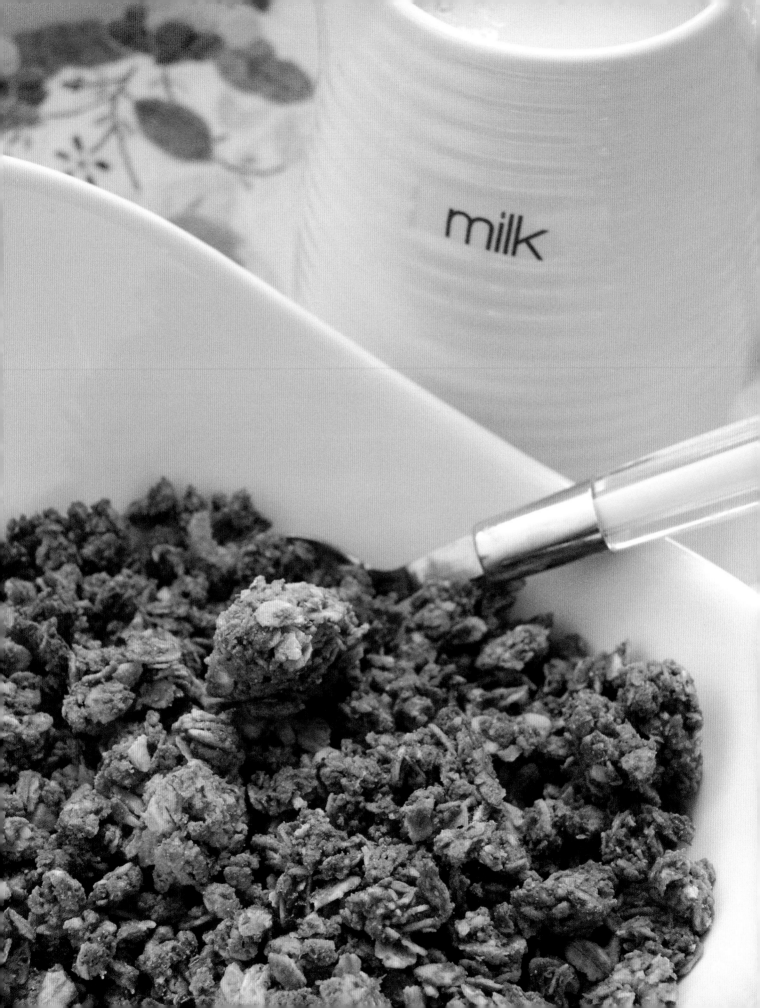
milk

Peanut Butter Coconut Quinoa Granola (vegan)
Makes 3 cups

ingredients
¼ cup and 2 Tablespoons natural peanut butter, warmed
2 cups gluten-free old-fashioned rolled oats
¼ teaspoon sea salt
½ teaspoon vanilla extract
¼ cup brown rice syrup
¼ cup unsweetened shredded coconut
2 Tablespoons flaxseed meal
¼ cup quinoa flakes

directions
Preheat oven at 300°F. Prepare a baking sheet by lining with parchment paper or baking mat. Soften peanut butter by scooping into a small, microwave-safe bowl and placing in microwave for about 10 seconds. You may also warm the peanut butter in a small pot over low heat, stirring constantly until soft.

In a medium bowl, combine the peanut butter, oats, sea salt ,vanilla extract, and brown rice syrup. Stir until ingredients are well combined. Add the coconut, flaxseed meal, and quinoa flakes, stirring until mixed thoroughly.

Spread the mixture onto the baking sheet and then bake in oven for 35–40 minutes, until golden brown. Toss the granola with a spatula halfway through the bake time.

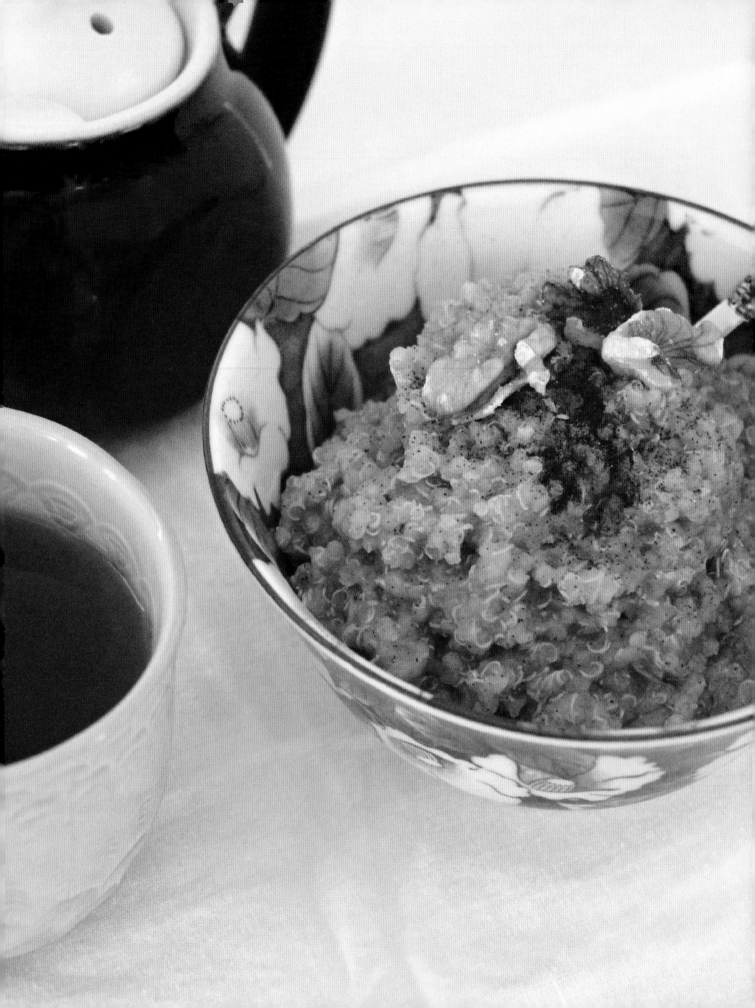

Banana Bread Quinoa Cereal (vegan)

Makes 2 servings

This is what I like to call a "sticks to the ribs" breakfast. When I am feeling extra hungry and a green smoothie or omelette just won't do, I whip up a bowl of this toasty cereal and enjoy it with a warm cup of tea. It makes me feel all snuggly inside.

ingredients
1¼ cups cooked quinoa
1 ripe banana
¼ cup pure maple syrup
⅓ dairy-free unsweetened vanilla milk
½ teaspoon ground cinnamon
⅛ teaspoon sea salt
⅓ cup raw walnuts, divided

directions
In a small pot, combine quinoa, banana, maple syrup, milk, cinnamon, and sea salt, warming over low-medium heat. Stir constantly, mashing banana against sides of pot to break up large pieces. Cook for 6–8 minutes, until warm and milk is absorbed. Divide walnuts among bowls, sprinkling on top. Serve and enjoy.

Quick Tip: Keep cooked quinoa and brown rice on hand, so that they can easily be tossed into recipes or served as a side.

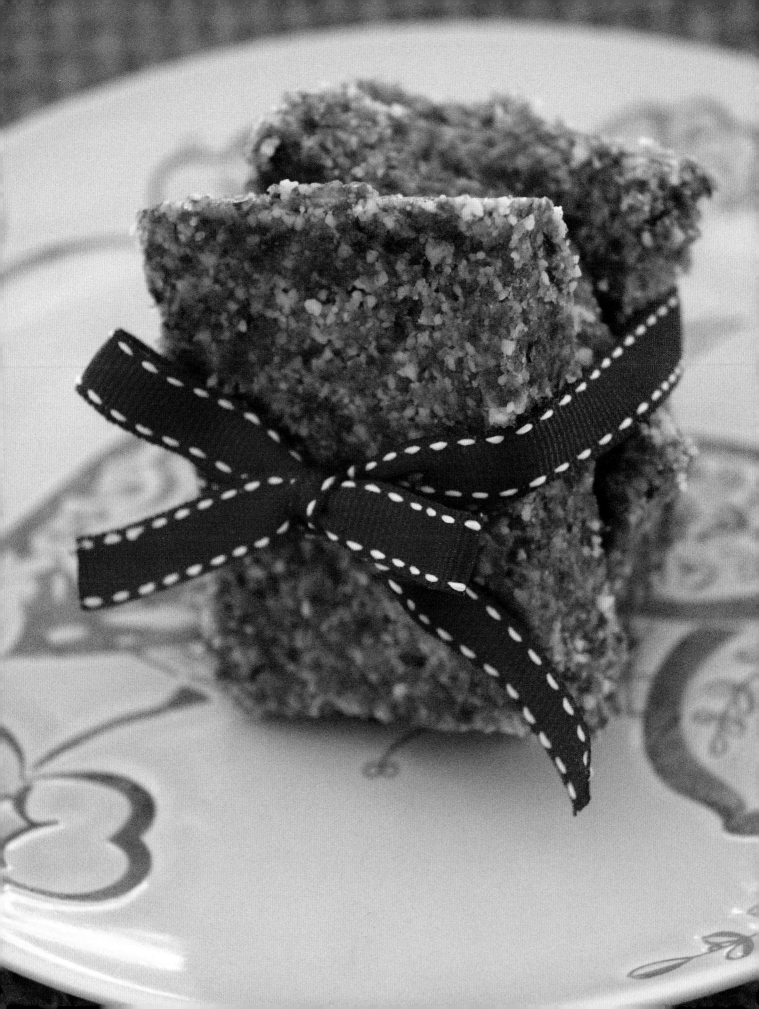

Raw Sour Cherry Almond Bar (vegan)

Makes 8 bars

Let's face it: Sometimes food bars are our go-to option when eating a solid meal just isn't going to happen. The downside, of course, is that they often cost a gajillion dollars, boasting a price tag that could score you a solid salad from the market. Save some dough by making these babies at home and keep 'em on hand for days when you need a quick snack.

ingredients

2½ cups raw almonds
⅓ cup dried sour cherries
1 cup dates, pits removed and chopped
⅓ cup shredded unsweetened coconut
1 teaspoon vanilla extract
¾ teaspoon sea salt
juice of ½ a lemon, seeds removed

directions

Pulse all ingredients in a food processor or high-speed blender until pulverized. Scoop mixture into a 9x9-inch square baking dish using a spatula to press into dish and spread evenly. Refrigerate for 1 hour and then cut into squares. Store bars in refrigerator.

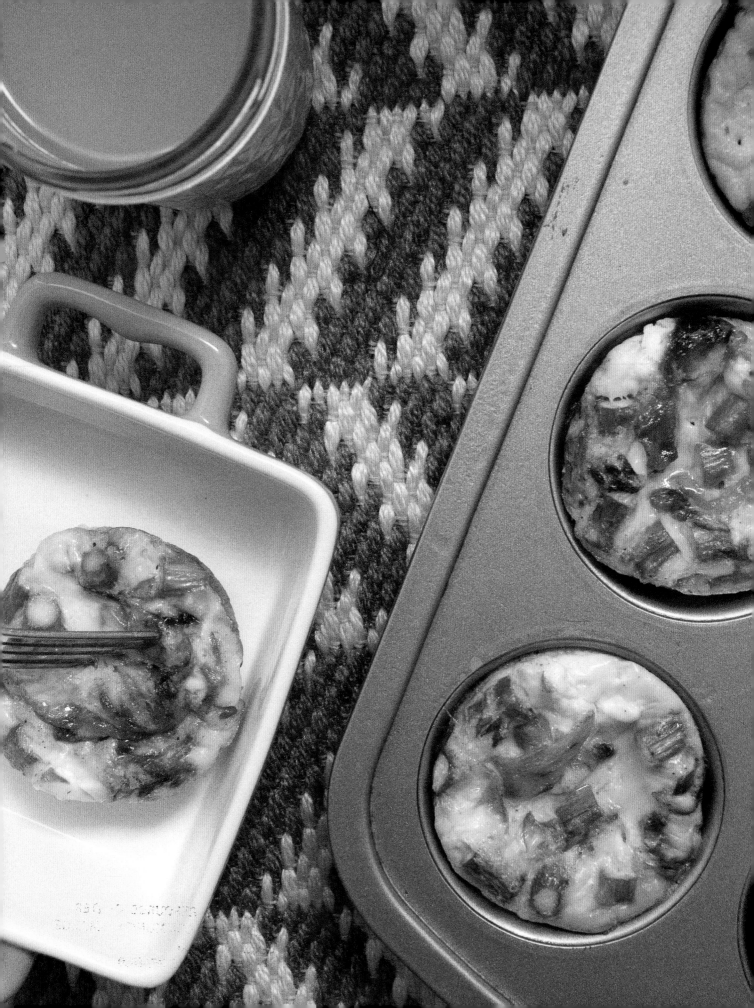

Goat Cheese & Asparagus Quiche Cups with Caramelized Onions (vegetarian)

Makes 12 servings

ingredients
6 large eggs
3 large egg whites
¼ cup of water
¼ teaspoon sea salt
⅛ teaspoon ground nutmeg
1 medium yellow onion, caramelized (see instructions on page 53)
1½ cups chopped fresh asparagus
4 ounces goat cheese, crumbled

directions
Preheat oven to 350°F. Prepare a 12-cup muffin pan by spraying with non-stick baking spray or brushing with oil. Set aside.

In a medium bowl, whisk together eggs, egg whites, water, sea salt, and nutmeg until combined. Pour egg mixture into each cup, filling about ¾ full.

Divide prepared caramelized onion, asparagus, and goat cheese evenly among muffin cups.

Place muffin pan in oven, baking for 18–20 minutes, until tops of quiche cups turn golden brown. Cool in pan for 5–8 minutes before running a butter knife along the sides of each cup to loosen. Serve and enjoy!

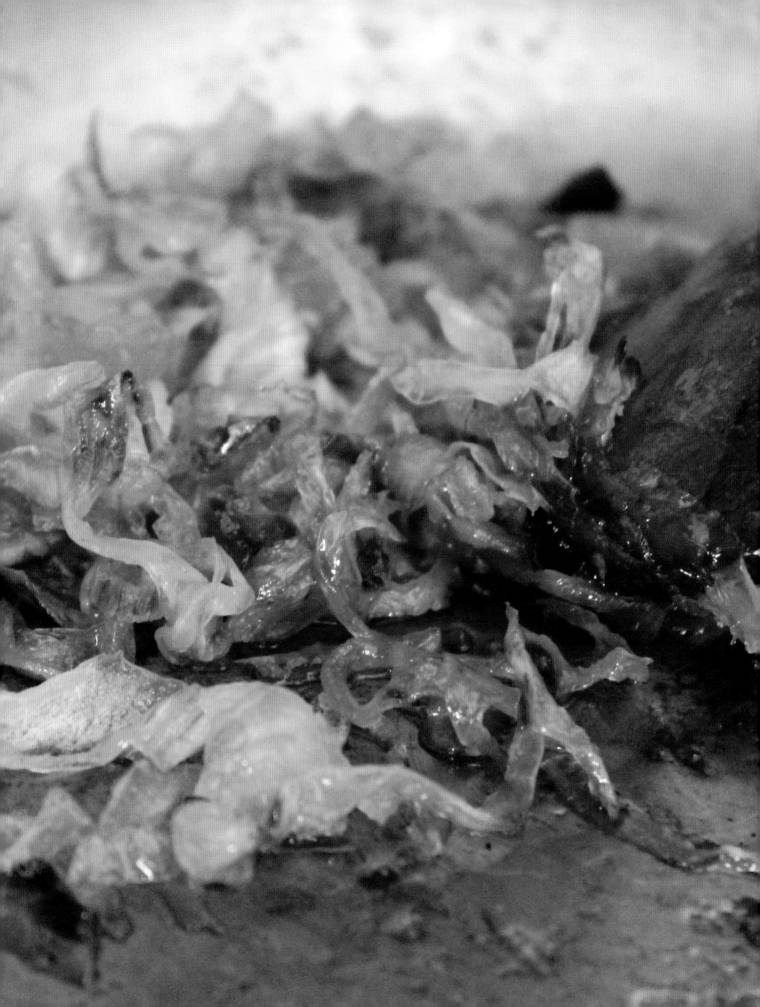

How to Caramelize an Onion

Caramelized onions are my jam. I love them on top of a veggie burger, stuffed inside an omelette or simply straight out of the pan. Want to make your house smell like heaven? Caramelize an onion. Want to do a my-belly-is-so-happy dance? Caramelize an onion. Like the idea of . . . okay, seriously, just caramelize an onion.

ingredients
3 Tablespoons salted butter
1 whole yellow onion, thinly sliced
¼ teaspoon sea salt
1 Tablespoon granulated sugar

directions
Heat butter in a medium pan over low heat. Add onion and sea salt, frequently stirring for 30 minutes. Sprinkle sugar on top of onion mixture, cooking for an additional 15 minutes, stirring consistently throughout. Remove from heat and serve.

Sweet Potato Spinach Quiche with Oatmeal Crust
(vegetarian)
Makes 8 servings

ingredients
1 prepared oatmeal crust (see page 145)
2 Tablespoons extra-virgin olive oil
2 garlic cloves, minced
½ medium sweet potato, cut into ¼-inch thick slices
6 large egg whites
2 large eggs
¼ cup shredded fresh baby spinach leaves
¼ teaspoon sea salt

directions
Preheat oven to 350°F. Press prepared oatmeal crust into an 8-inch pie pan until evenly distributed. Set aside.

Heat olive oil in a medium pan over low-medium heat. Add garlic and sweet potato slices, cooking for 5–6 minutes, until browned. Flip potato slices halfway through cook time to ensure even browning. Remove from heat and set aside.

In a medium bowl, whisk together eggs, egg whites, spinach, and sea salt. Layer potato slices on bottom of oatmeal crust, overlapping if necessary. Pour egg mixture on top of slices, then place in oven for 30 minutes, or until browned on top and center has set. Allow quiche to cool for 5 minutes before slicing and serving.

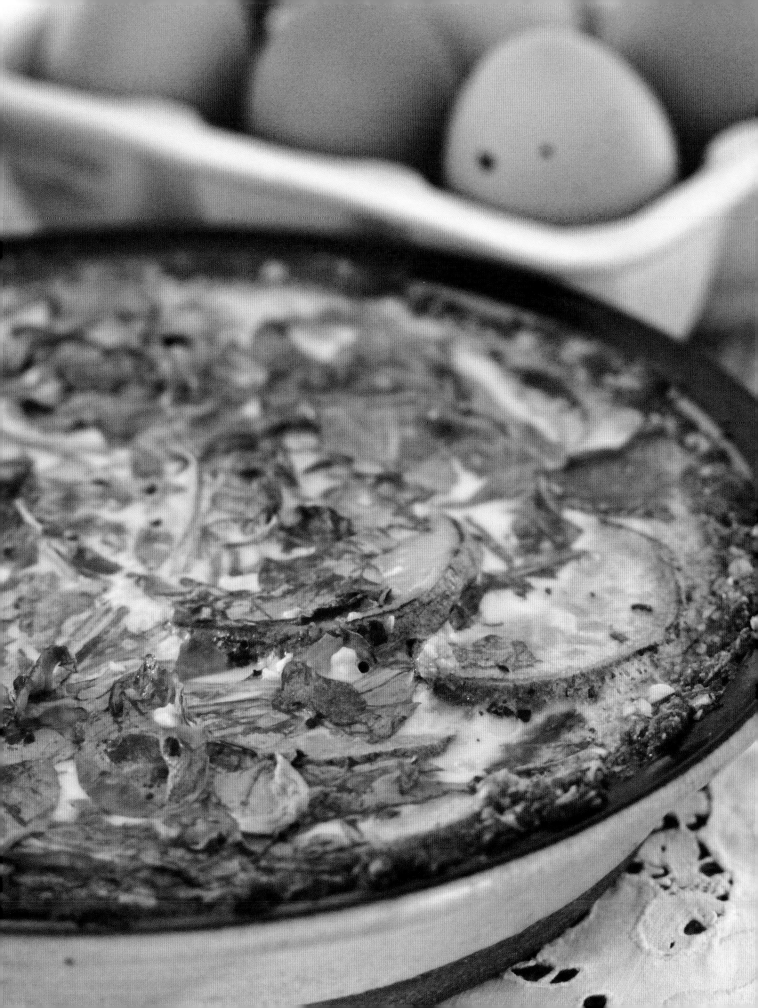

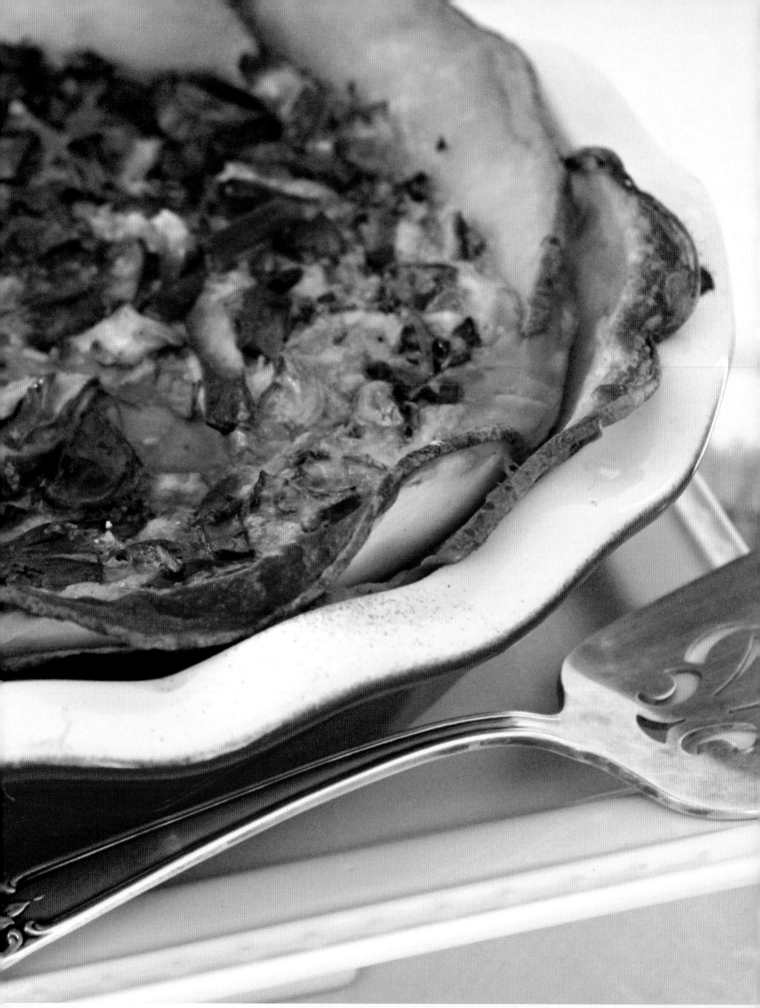

Mushroom Potato Crust Quiche (vegetarian)

Makes 8 servings

ingredients

1 russet potato, cut into ¼-inch thick slices
6 large eggs
3 large egg whites
¼ teaspoon sea salt
1 Tablespoon water
3 ounces baby portabella mushrooms, rinsed and sliced
½ cup shredded cheddar cheese
2 garlic cloves, minced
extra-virgin olive oil, for brushing

directions

Preheat oven to 325°F. Line a 9-inch pie pan with potato slices, overlapping when necessary. Some edges of potatoes will extend beyond the edge of pie pan. Set aside.

In a medium bowl, whisk together eggs, egg whites, sea salt, and water. Stir in mushrooms, cheddar cheese, and garlic. Pour mixture into potato-lined pie dish. Brush exposed potato edges with olive oil, using a silicone basting brush.

Place quiche into oven and bake for 50–52 minutes, until center has set. Allow it to cool for 5 minutes before slicing and serving.

NOTE: A good test for "doneness" with this or any quiche is that the center does not wobble when lightly tapped with finger.

Want to spice things up? Add your favorite herb, like sage, thyme, or rosemary, to the egg mixture.

Raspberry Lemonade Doughnuts (vegan)

Makes 12 doughnuts

ingredients
cake

2 flaxseed eggs (2 Tablespoons flaxseed meal, plus 6 Tablespoons warm water)
1 cup granulated vegan sugar
½ cup unsweetened applesauce
¼ cup and 2 Tablespoons grapeseed or safflower oil
juice and zest of ½ fresh lemon, seeds removed
½ cup fresh raspberries
2 cups Gluten-Free All-Purpose Baking Mix (see recipe on page 144)
1 teaspoon baking powder
½ teaspoon baking soda
¼ teaspoon sea salt

glaze

2 Tablespoons unsweetened vanilla dairy-free milk
¼ teaspoon pure vanilla extract
1 cup powdered sugar

directions
For cake

Preheat oven to 325°F. Prepare doughnut pan by brushing with oil or using a non-stick spray. Mix together the flaxseed meal and water in a small bowl and allow it to sit for a few minutes.

Combine flour, baking powder, baking soda, cinnamon, and sea salt in a medium bowl and set aside.

Using a standing mixer or medium bowl with hand mixer, combine vegan sugar, applesauce, grapeseed oil, lemon juice, and lemon zest. Add flaxseed eggs, then raspberries, mixing on low-medium speed. Slowly add flour combination to the wet ingredients, mixing until combined. Fill each doughnut cup ¾ full. Bake for 30–35 minutes until golden brown, or until a toothpick inserted toward the center comes out clean. Allow doughnuts to sit in pan for 6–8 minutes, then transfer to a baking rack to cool completely.

For glaze:
While doughnuts are cooling, combine milk, vanilla extract, and powdered sugar in a small pot. Place over low heat and begin continuously whisking. Continue this process until all lumps have dissolved. Remove from heat.

Dip one side of each doughnut in the glaze, then place back on the wire baking rack to set. Repeat until all doughnuts have been coated.

NOTE: Place a tray or parchment paper under the wire rack to catch excess glaze that will drip from doughnuts.

Tip No time for doughnuts? Preheat the oven to 350°F and place the batter in a greased 9x5-inch loaf pan to make a quick bread instead. Bake for 70–75 minutes (until a toothpick comes out clean), then drizzle glaze on top.

dressings, marinades & toppings

Honey Mustard Dressing
Traditional Balsamic Vinaigrette
Lemon Garlic Cleansing Dressing
Sesame Marinade
Roasted Walnut Herb Pesto
Sweet & Sour Caponata

Like chips & dip or Bonnie & Clyde, some matches are simply meant to be. Whip up these dressings and toppings to spice up a dish or add a new spin to an old favorite.

Honey Mustard Dressing

Makes 2 servings

ingredients
2 Tablespoons extra-virgin olive oil
2 teaspoons Dijon mustard
1 teaspoon honey
½ teaspoon red wine vinegar
1 teaspoon minced garlic
½ teaspoon chopped thyme

directions
Mix all ingredients together until combined.

Get creative: Swap honey for equal parts agave nectar to make this dressing vegan.

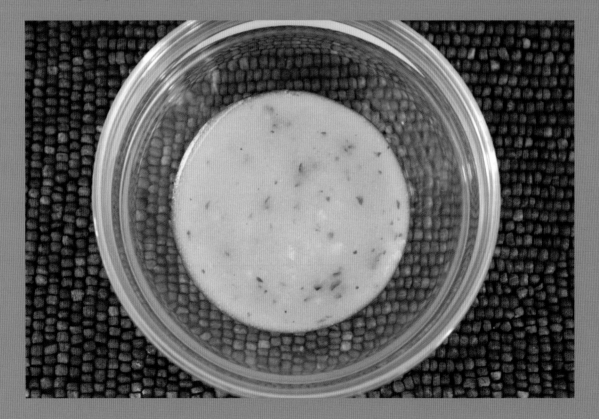

How to Pair Greens & Dressings

Discover various types of lettuces, then match them to the dressings on the following pages.

Boston & Bibb Lettuces: Subtle and buttery (just like the name indicates), these lettuces pair well with a simple balsamic vinaigrette.

Radicchio and Arugula: Both are peppery and perfect with Boston & Bibb lettuces or spinach. These lettuces are great with a honey mustard dressing.

Spinach: This iron-packed green is tasty with a citrus vinaigrette, like the Lemon Garlic Cleansing Dressing (see page 65).

Romaine: Packed with calcium, this sweet leafy veggie is yummy, rather versatile, and pairs well with most dressings.

Traditional Balsamic Vinaigrette

Makes 2 servings

ingredients
3 Tablespoons extra-virgin olive oil
2 teaspoons balsamic vinegar
1 teaspoon Dijon mustard
1 teaspoon minced garlic or shallot
1 teaspoon finely chopped thyme (optional)

directions
Mix all ingredients together until combined.

Get creative: Try one of your favorite herbs, like oregano or rosemary, in place of the thyme.

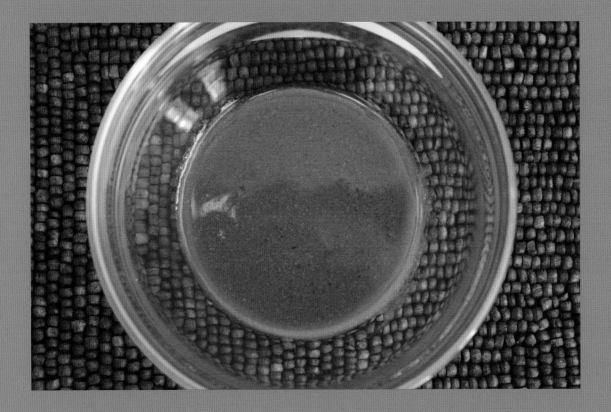

Lemon Garlic Cleansing Dressing
Makes 2 servings

ingredients
3 Tablespoons extra virgin olive oil
1 Tablespoon chopped parsley
2 garlic cloves, minced
juice of 1 lemon, seeds removed

directions
Mix all ingredients together until combined.

Get creative: Out of lemons? Try lime for an equally zippy kick!

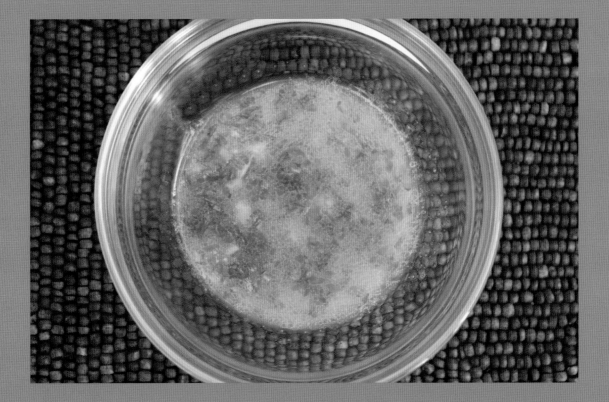

Sesame Marinade

Makes 1 serving

ingredients
2 Tablespoons extra-virgin olive oil
1 garlic clove, minced
1 teaspoon minced ginger
2 teaspoons tamari
1 teaspoon Dijon mustard
1 teaspoon honey
1 teaspoon toasted sesame oil

directions
Mix all ingredients together until combined.

Nori-Wrapped Fish or Tofu: Use Your Leftovers

Use the Sesame Marinade (see page 66) to spice up a fresh piece of wild caught fish or slice of extra-firm tofu. Simply whisk the marinade ingredients together, then place it in a resealable bag with tofu or fish, and allow it to marinate for 30 minutes.

Cook the fish or tofu in a sauté pan, or grill it on a warm summer day. You can serve the fish or tofu solo, or place it between two nori sheets along with any lettuce and veggies you have on hand (try leftover **Brown Sugar Glazed Carrots & Parsnips** featured on page 95), then wrap it up like a burrito. Enjoy!

Roasted Walnut Herb Pesto

Makes 1½ cups

ingredients
1 cup walnuts
2 cups herbs of choice (e.g., rosemary, sage, basil, thyme, and/or oregano)
3 garlic cloves
2 Tablespoons extra-virgin olive oil
¼ teaspoon sea salt

directions
Preheat oven to 350°F. Place walnuts on a small baking sheet and roast for 5–6 minutes. Remove from oven and allow to cool for 5 minutes.

   Add walnuts, herbs, garlic, olive oil, and sea salt to a food processor. Mix until smooth.

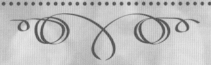

Sweet & Sour Caponata: Use Your Leftovers

Save a bit of your leftover Sloppy Faux Joes mix (see page 130) for this caponata, best served over grilled tofu or fish.

ingredients
1 cup leftover Sloppy Faux Joes
1½ Tablespoons pine nuts
¼ cup raisins
½ cup pitted and chopped black and green olives
ground pepper and sea salt, to taste

directions
Combine all ingredients in a medium pot over low-medium heat. Simmer for 6–8 minutes, stirring throughout. Serve over prepared tofu or fish.

just a bite

Open-Faced Polenta Caprese Sandwiches
Curried Chickpea Bites
Sweet Potato French Fry Dip
Ginger Sesame Seed Cucumbers
Black Bean & Banana Salsa
Snails & Seeds Dinner Rolls
Stuffed Mini Red Potatoes
Asian-Infused Lettuce Wraps

Whether you simply need a little nosh, or you are playing the role of hostess, these small dishes will keep your belly feeling happy while you wait for the main event.

Open-Faced Polenta Caprese Sandwiches
Makes 16 servings

ingredients
1 24-ounce package of polenta, sliced
¼ cup extra-virgin olive oil
1 Tablespoon minced fresh sage
1 Tablespoon minced fresh oregano
1 Tablespoon minced fresh thyme
¼ teaspoon sea salt
1 8-ounce package of buffalo mozzarella cheese
1 cup grape or cherry tomatoes, sliced
16 fresh basil leaves
Traditional Balsamic Vinaigrette (see page 64)
ground pepper, as desired

directions
Preheat oven at 350°F. Line a baking sheet with parchment paper or baking mat. Arrange polenta slices on the paper or mat.

In a small bowl, mix olive oil, sage, oregano, thyme, and sea salt. Using a silicone brush, spread olive oil mixture on top of each slice. Place in oven and bake for 25–30 minutes, until golden brown. Remove from oven and allow polenta to cool until warm.

Top each polenta slice with mozzarella, a basil leaf, and 3–4 tomato slices each. Drizzle with balsamic dressing and ground pepper as desired.

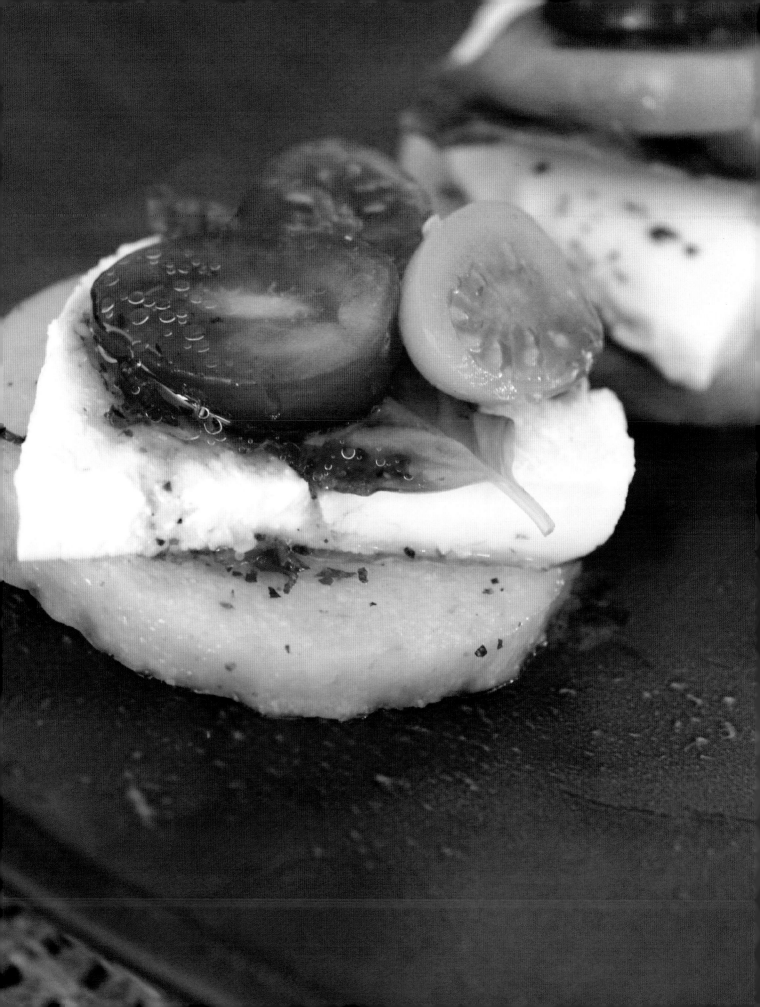

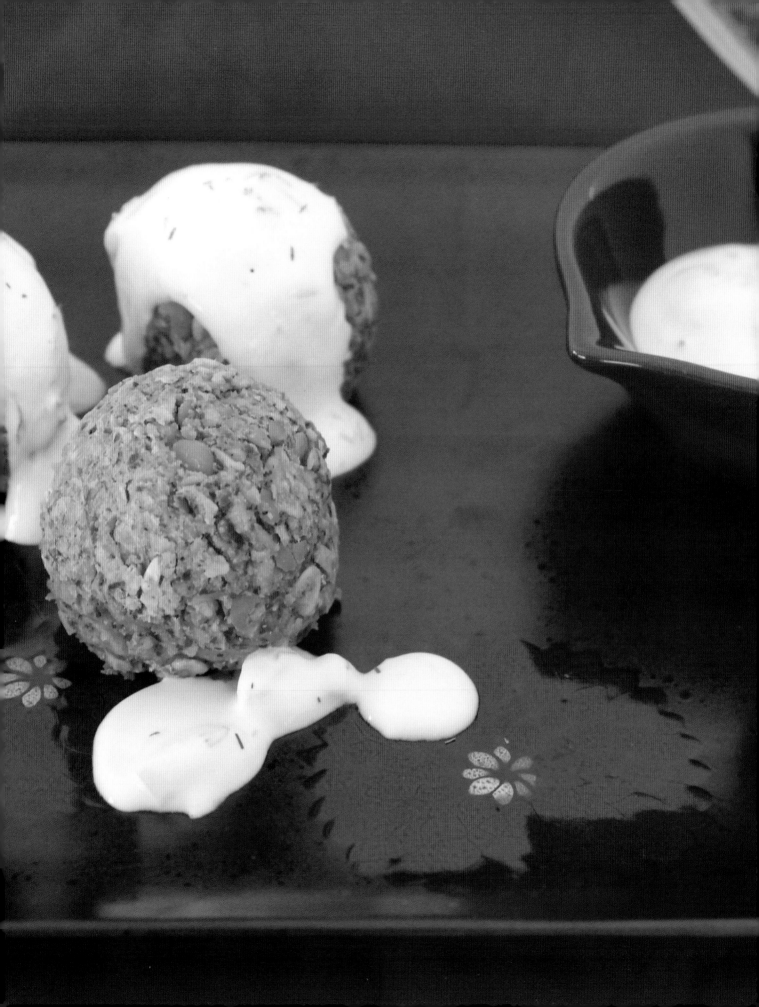

Curried Chickpea Bites with Cucumber Dill Sauce
(vegan option)
Makes 12 bites

bites
2 Tablespoons extra-virgin olive oil, plus extra for brushing
2 cups diced sweet potato
¼ medium onion, diced
1 14.5-ounce can chickpeas
2–3 garlic cloves, minced
¼ teaspoon garam masala spice
½ teaspoon sea salt
¾ teaspoon curry powder
2 flaxseed eggs (2 Tablespoons flaxseed meal, plus 6 Tablespoons warm water)

sauce
1 cup sour cream (regular or vegan)
1 Tablespoon minced fresh dill
2 Tablespoons diced cucumbers
¼ teaspoon sea salt

directions
Preheat oven to 350°F. Prepare a baking pan by lining it with parchment paper or baking mat.

In a small bowl, combine flaxseed meal and water, then set aside. Sauté olive oil, sweet potatoes and onions in a large skillet over medium heat, stirring occasionally. Allow mixture to cool for ten minutes.

Add flaxseed meal mixture, sweet potato mixture, and remaining ingredients to a food processor. Pulse until mixture is combined, but not smooth (portions of sweet potato and chickpeas will still be visible). Using hands, shape the mixture into 12 balls, placing each one on the prepared baking pan.

Bake for 40–42 minutes, until the balls begin to turn golden brown.

While the chickpea bites are baking, prepare the sauce, adding all ingredients to a medium bowl and stirring until well combined. Keep refrigerated until ready to serve.

Sweet Potato French Fry Dip (vegan)

Makes 2½ cups

You might have a tough time getting your little one to eat a whole sweet potato, but this dip is a great way to make sure they get that healthy dose of one of nature's best sources of beta-carotene. The best part? The kiddos will eat it up, but the diners at the big kids table will love it, too. Serve with veggies or gluten-free crackers and you're good-to-go.

ingredients

2½ cups unseasoned sweet potato french fries, prepared according to package and cooled
½ cup canned chickpeas, rinsed and drained
2 garlic cloves
2 Tablespoons extra-virgin olive oil
¼ teaspoon sea salt
¼ teaspoon chili powder
2–3 Tablespoons cold water (to loosen)

directions

Place prepared french fries, chickpeas, garlic cloves, olive oil, sea salt, and chili powder into a food processor. Pulse until smooth. If mixture is too thick, then add cold water, 1 Tablespoon at a time. Refrigerate in resealable container until serving.

NOTE: Don't have sweet potato fries on hand? Use the real thing by dicing up 2½ cups of fresh sweet potatoes, setting the oven to 400°F and roasting them until soft (about 35 minutes). Allow them to cool, then follow the recipe directions accordingly!

Why beta-carotene? The nutrients in a sweet potato are ideal for maintaining a healthy immune system and superb vision. Same goes for dark leafy greens, broccoli, and carrots. Plus, the addition of a little bit of fat—in this case, olive oil—helps you reap the maximum benefits of this power-packed root veggie!

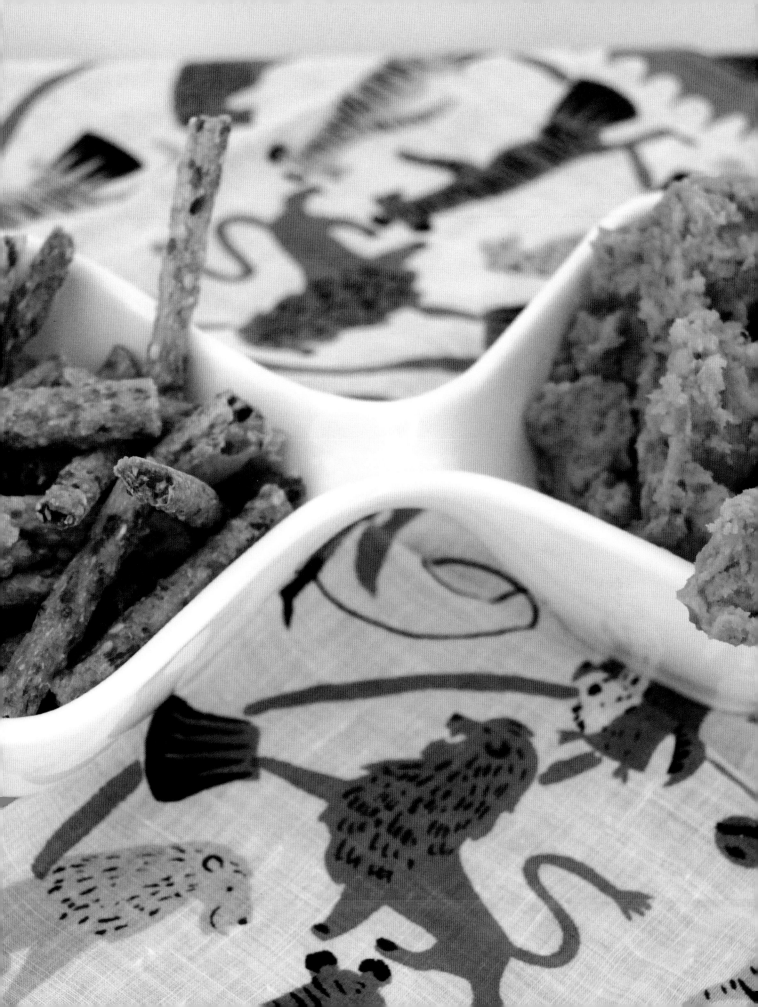

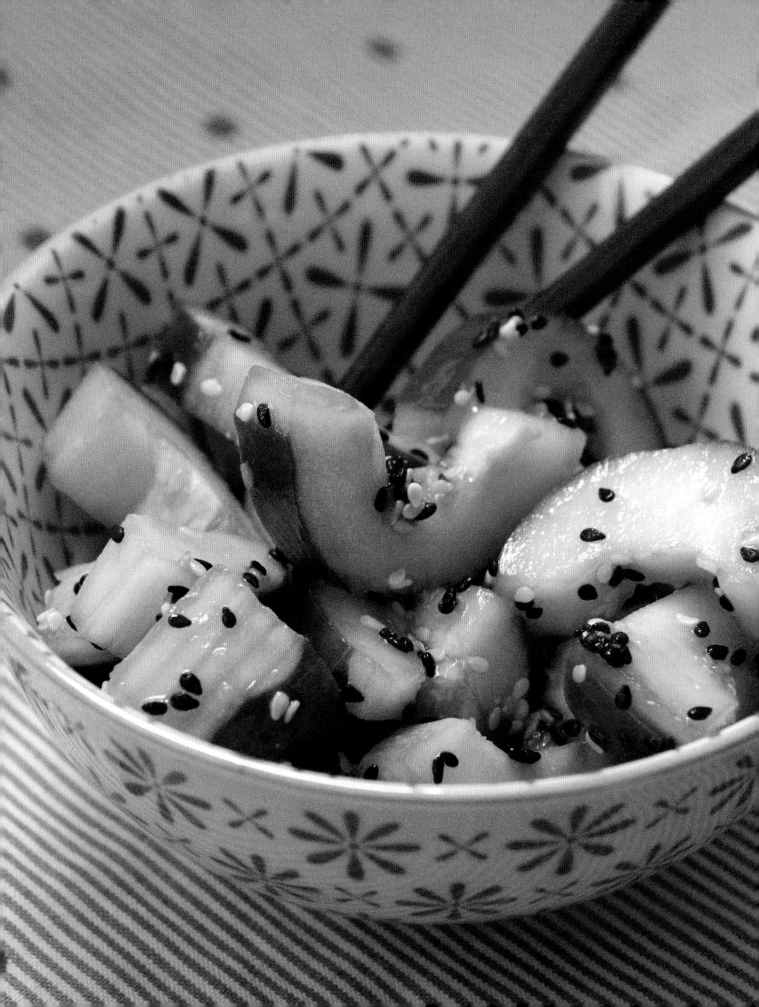

Ginger Sesame Seed Cucumbers

Makes 2–3 servings

Serve these cucumbers cold and pair them with fresh grilled fish or as an appetizer to a meal. They are so simple to make and simply delightful!

ingredients

1 medium organic cucumber, peeled lengthwise in strips
2 Tablespoons tamari
1 teaspoon mirin rice cooking wine
1 teaspoon minced ginger
2 Tablespoons sesame seeds (white or black)
½ teaspoon toasted sesame oil

directions

Prepare cucumber by slicing lengthwise and removing seeds. Cut each half into slices and set aside.

In a medium bowl, mix tamari, mirin, ginger, sesame seeds, and sesame oil. Drizzle over cucumbers and toss to serve.

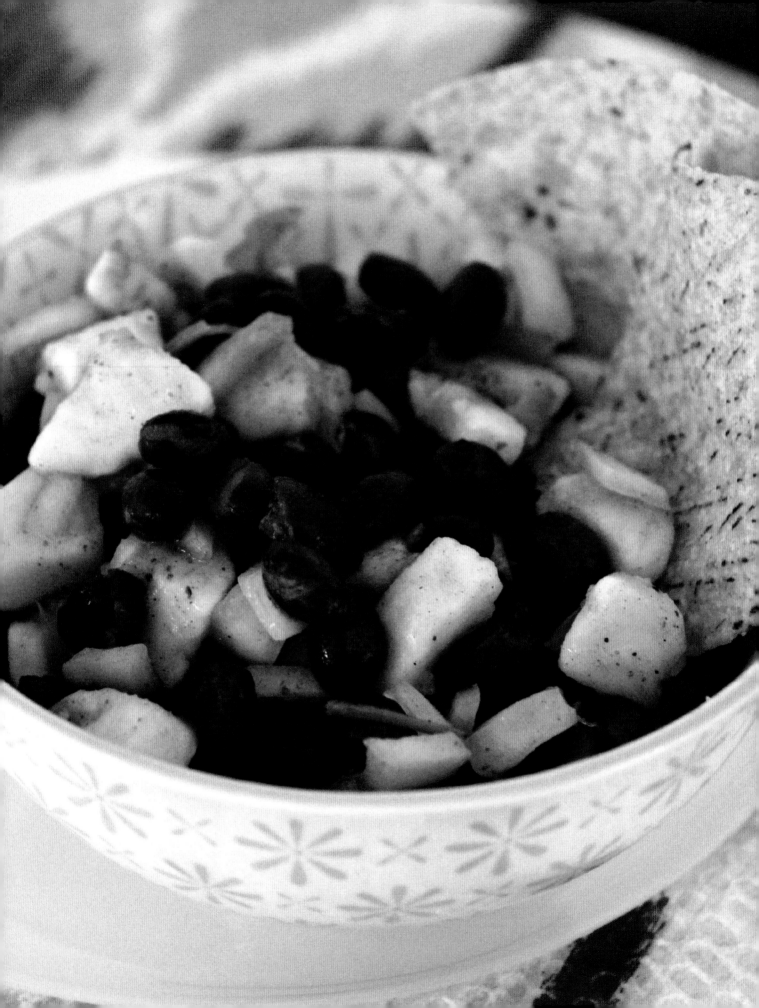

Black Bean & Banana Salsa (vegan)

Makes 3½ cups

This dip is like a fiesta for your belly. Enjoy with gluten-free crackers or chips.

ingredients

1 15-ounce can black beans, rinsed and drained
1 ripe banana, cubed
⅓ cup yellow onion, diced
2 Tablespoons fresh cilantro, minced
1 garlic clove, minced
juice of 1 fresh lime
⅛ teaspoon sea salt
¼ teaspoon chili powder

directions

In a medium bowl, combine all ingredients, mixing thoroughly. Refrigerate until ready to serve.

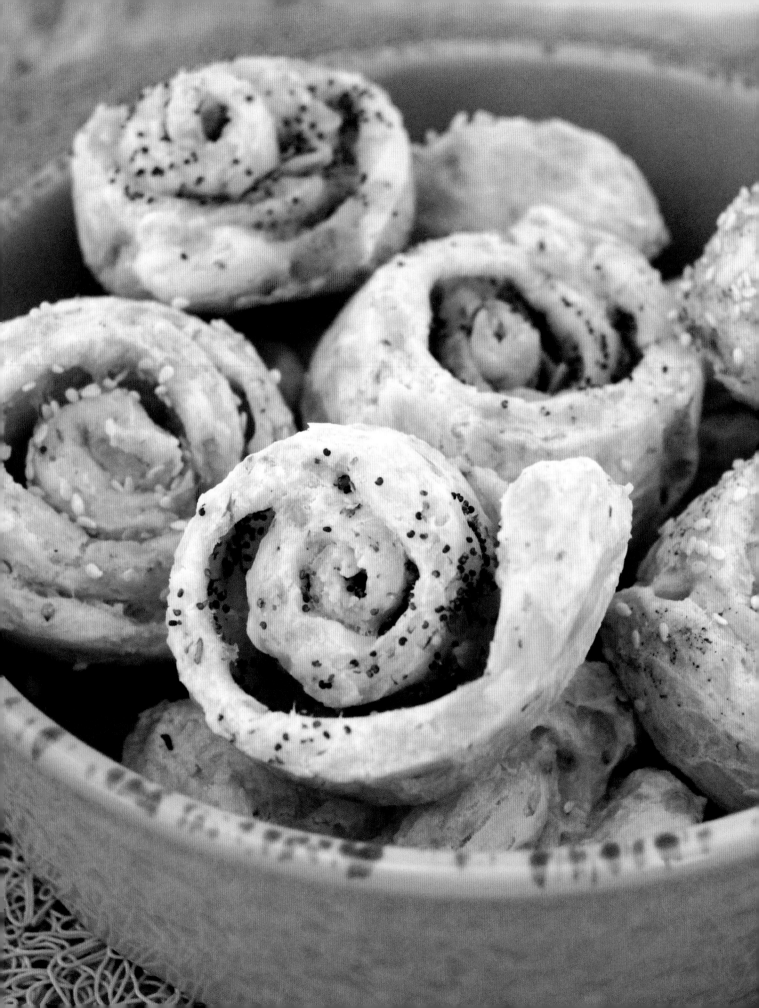

Snails & Seeds Dinner Rolls: Family Kitchen Fun
Makes 10–12 rolls

Get kids involved in the kitchen by preparing this dough ahead of time then allowing them to shape it into fun dinner rolls.

ingredients
8 ounces gluten-free bread dough mix, prepared and refrigerated for at least 2
   hours
1 Tablespoon poppy seeds
2 Tablespoons sesame seeds
¼ teaspoon paprika
gluten-free flour, for dusting

directions

Preheat oven to 350°F. Prepare a baking sheet by lining with parchment paper or baking mat, then set aside.

Place parchment paper down on a work surface, securing each end with masking tape or heavy objects that will keep it from sliding. Dust surface with gluten-free flour, then place bread dough in center.

Dust a rolling pin with gluten-free flour, then begin to roll out bread dough until evenly ¼-inch thick. Slice into vertical strips about 1½ inches wide.

In a small bowl, mix together poppy seeds, sesame seeds, paprika, and sea salt. Sprinkle each strip with mixture, then roll from one end to other to form "snail." Place on prepared baking sheet and continue until all strips are completed.

Bake for 18–20 minutes, or until rolls turn golden brown. (Actual baking time may vary depending on bread mix you choose.)

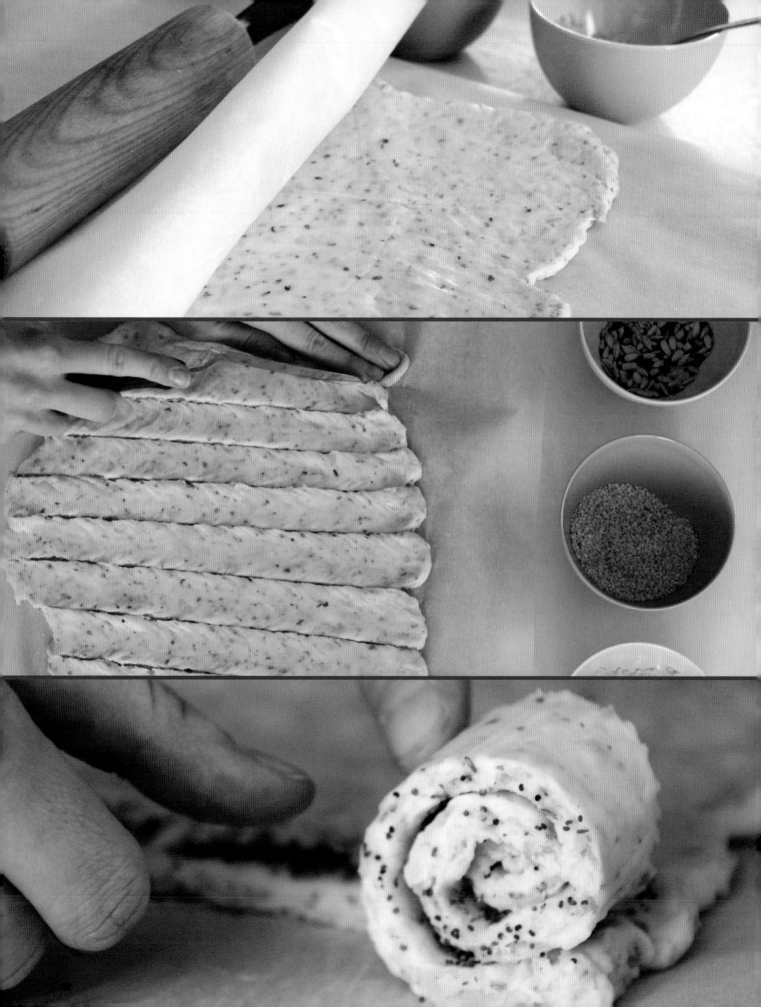

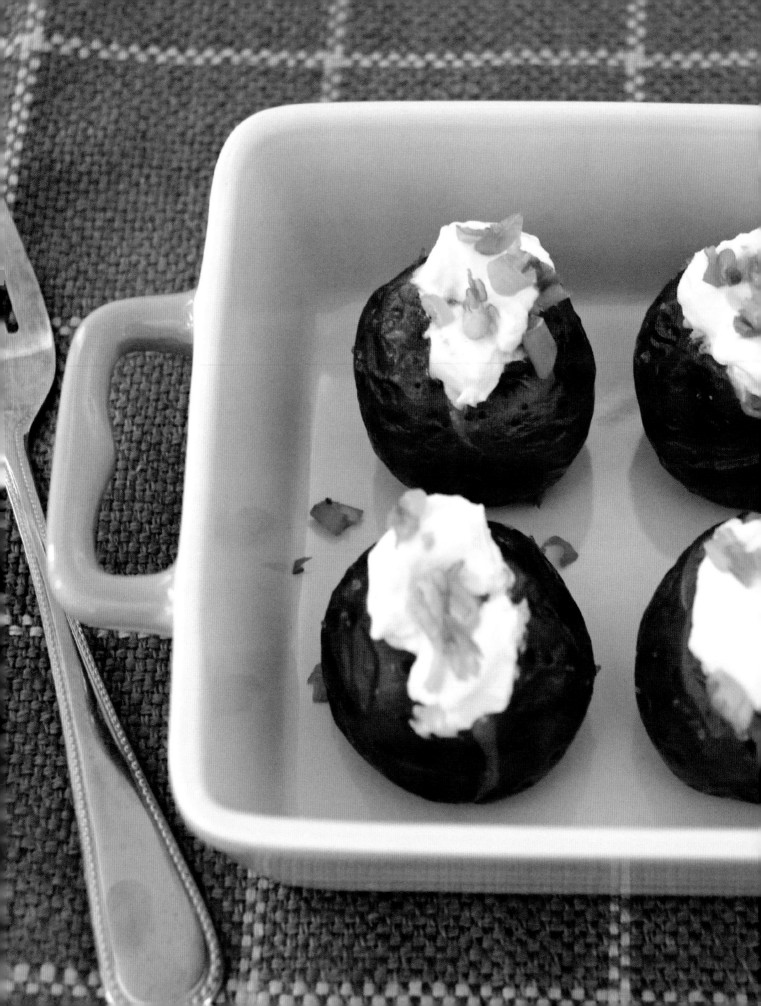

Stuffed Mini Red Potatoes (vegan option)

Makes about 25 potatoes

ingredients

1½ lbs of petite red potatoes
2 Tablespoons extra-virgin olive oil
sea salt, to taste
2 Tablespoons butter (regular or vegan)
¼ cup and 2 Tablespoons sour cream (regular or vegan)
chives, minced (as desired)

directions

Preheat oven to 450°F. Place potatoes on a large cookie sheet, using a silicone brush to coat with olive oil. Sprinkle sea salt on potatoes. Bake for 25 minutes, or until a fork can easily pierce through the center of the potato.

Remove potatoes from oven and allow to cool for five minutes. Using a butter knife, cut a 1-inch slit in the top of each potato. Squeeze the ends of potato to open up the center a bit. Place about ¼ teaspoon butter into each potato, then top with 1 teaspoon of sour cream. Sprinkle with chives and serve.

Asian-Infused Lettuce Wraps
Makes 5–6 wraps

2 teaspoons mirin rice cooking wine
3 Tablespoons light brown sugar
4 Tablespoons tamari
½ teaspoon ground mustard
½ teaspoon toasted sesame oil
2 Tablespoons extra-virgin olive oil
4 Tablespoons pine nuts
2 cups cauliflower rice (see page 123)
2 cups shredded green cabbage
½ cup diced red pepper
5–6 Boston lettuce leaves
4 Tablespoons chopped green onions, divided
4 Tablespoons hemp seed, divided

directions

Combine mirin, brown sugar, tamari, ground mustard, and sesame oil in a small bowl, then set aside.

Add olive oil to a medium sauté pan, heating over low-medium heat, add pine nuts, cauliflower rice, green cabbage, and red pepper. Pour in mirin mixture, sautéing for 5–6 minutes and stirring occasionally. Remove from heat.

Prepare lettuce leaves on plates, then divide mixture among them. Sprinkle with green onions and hemp seed, then serve.

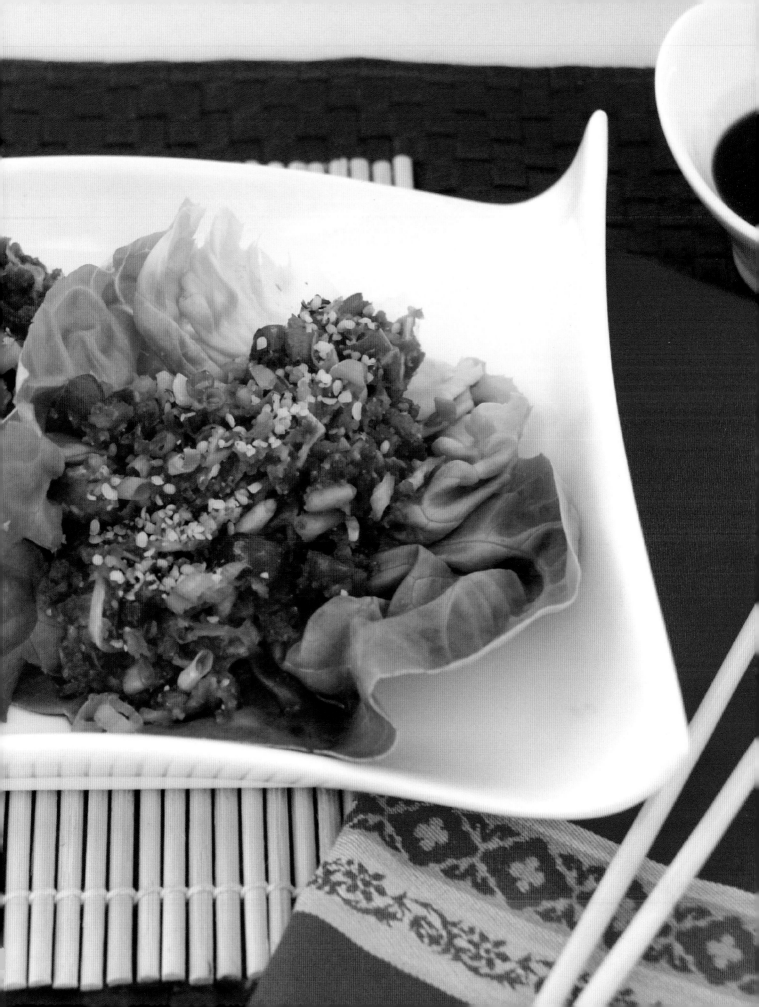

salads & sides

Rainbow Quinoa Salad
Brown Sugar–Glazed Carrots & Parsnips
Purifying Beet & Cabbage Salad
Grapefruit & Asparagus Salad
Black-Eyed Pea Quinoa Salad

In my opinion, the best salads and sides are those that can also stand on their own. In fact, one of my favorite quick dinner solutions is a mashup of leftover sides, all piled onto one plate!

Side dishes are an opportunity to create a balanced meal. Getting naughty with the Cheesy Tuna Tater Pie on page 112? Infuse some veggies into the mix by adding a helping of the Brown Sugar Glazed Carrots & Parsnips or Rainbow Quinoa Salad.

Rainbow Quinoa Salad

Makes 6–7 cups

This is another recipe where prepared quinoa kept in the refrigerator will come in handy. Serve at a lunch party or pair it with half a gluten-free sandwich for a yummy lunch option.

ingredients

2 cups cooked quinoa
1 cup canned garbanzo beans
1 cup diced celery
1 cup fresh blueberries
1 cup diced mixed bell peppers (red, yellow, orange)
½ cup diced green onions
½ cup chopped raw cashews
2 Tablespoons hemp seed
1 teaspoon garam masala
¼ cup apple cider vinegar
¼ cup extra-virgin olive oil
2 Tablespoons honey or agave syrup

directions

In a small bowl, whisk together apple cider vinegar, garam masala, olive oil, and honey. Set aside.

In a medium bowl, combine quinoa, garbanzo beans, celery, blueberries, peppers, green onions, cashews, and hemp seed, stirring to combine. Drizzle with apple cider vinegar mixture and toss before serving.

Tip! Rinse and drain quinoa before cooking to remove saponin, a coating that gives quinoa a bitter, soap-like taste.

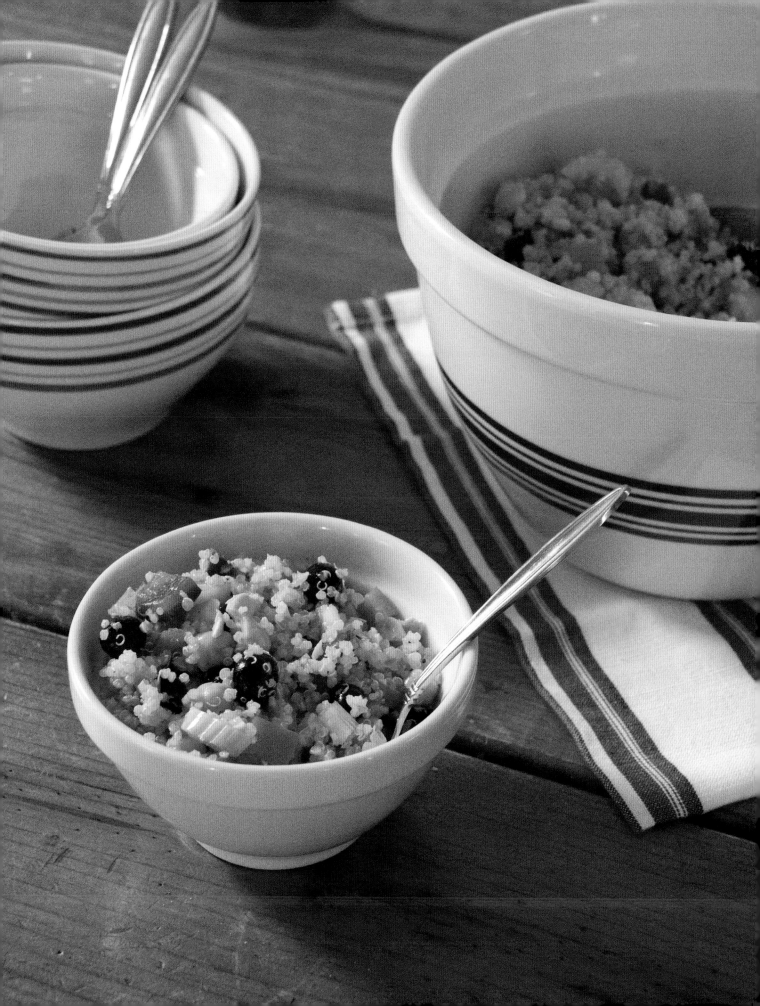

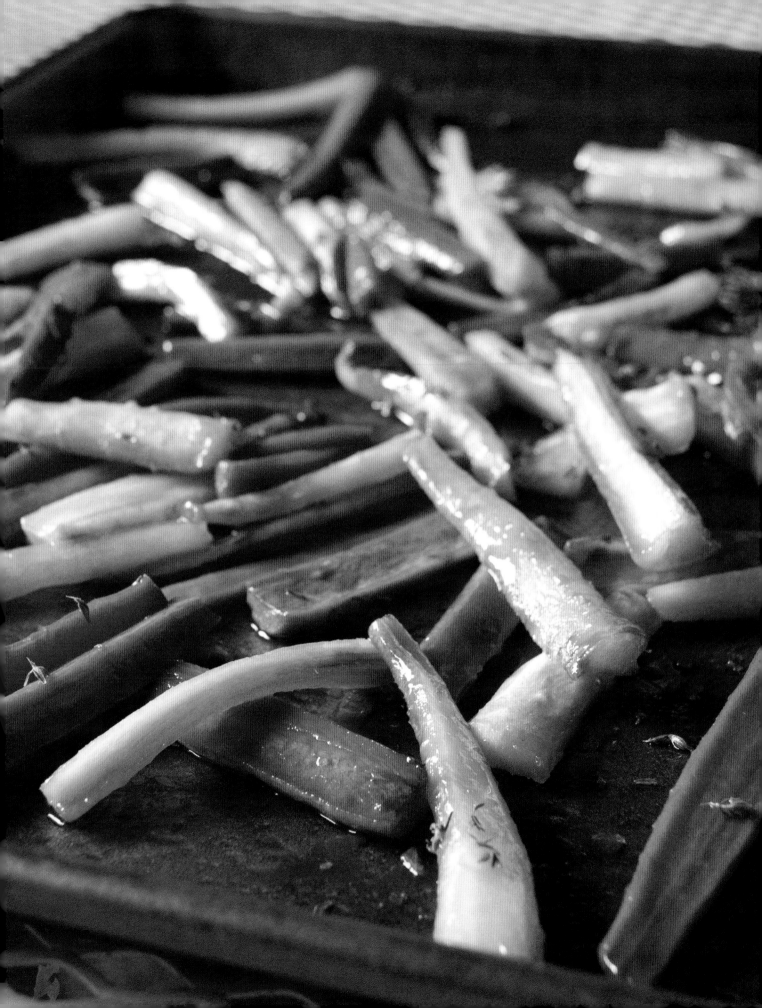

Brown Sugar–Glazed Carrots & Parsnips (vegan)
Makes 4 servings

ingredients
vegetables
6 fresh medium carrots
6 fresh medium parsnips
1 Tablespoon extra-virgin olive oil

topping
¼ cup vegan butter substitute
⅓ cup light brown sugar, packed
½ teaspoon sea salt
1 tablespoon minced fresh thyme

directions
Preheat oven to 400°F. Peel carrots and parsnips, then cut into ¼-inch thick sticks.

Place on a baking sheet and drizzle with olive oil. Roast for 15 minutes.

While carrots and parsnips are roasting, melt butter in a small saucepan, slowly adding brown sugar and sea salt. Stir until smooth, then remove from heat.

At 15 minutes cook time, remove vegetables from oven (don't forget to protect your hands!) and drizzle with brown sugar glaze. Roast for an additional 10 minutes. Remove from oven and toss with thyme. Serve immediately.

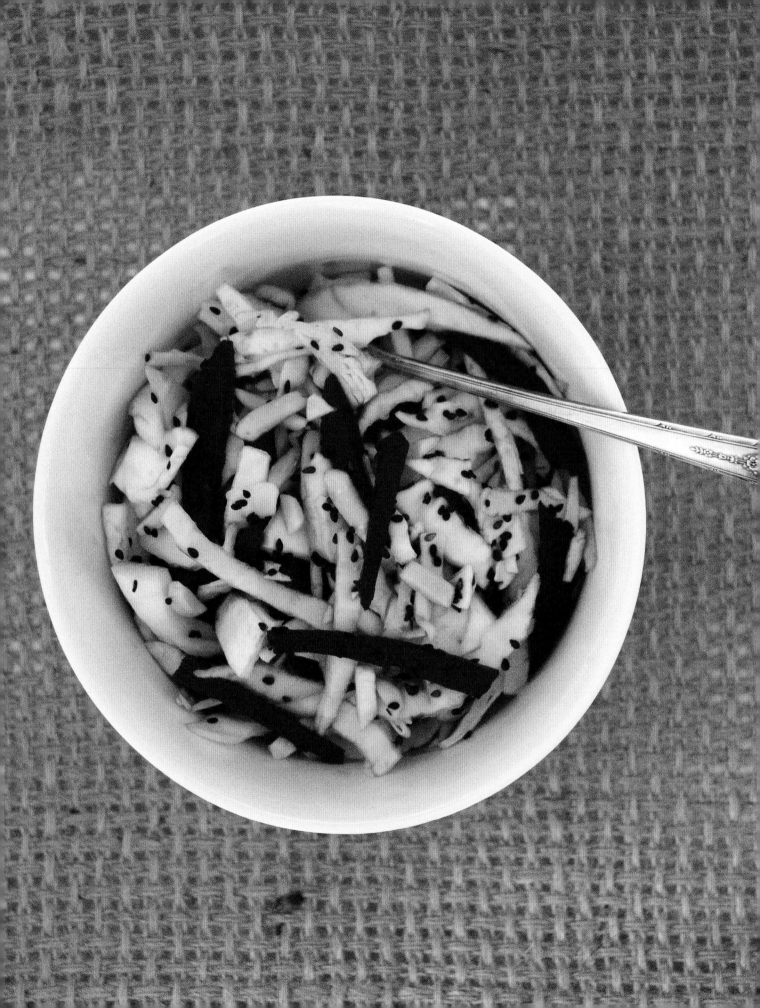

Purifying Beet & Cabbage Salad

Makes about 3 cups

Just like the Beet-iful Ginger Apple Smoothie (see page 36), this recipe is packed with vibrant nutrients. Pair it with fiber-rich cabbage for this simple and filling salad.

ingredients

1½ cups shredded green cabbage
1 cup thinly sliced cooked beets
¼ cup slivered raw almonds
2 Tablespoons black sesame seeds
2 Tablespoons mirin rice cooking wine
1 Tablespoon light brown sugar

directions

In a small bowl, combine mirin and brown sugar, breaking up brown sugar lumps by pressing against the sides of bowl with a fork. Set aside.

In a medium bowl, combine cabbage, beets, almonds, and sesame seeds. Drizzle mirin mixture on top and toss to combine. Store in refrigerator until ready to serve.

NOTE: Don't have black sesame seeds? Trade 'em for good ol' sesame seeds and turn out a yummy variation of the dish.

Grapefruit & Asparagus Salad with Parmesan Cheese and Balsamic Vinaigrette (vegan option)

Makes 2 servings

Half the beauty of this salad lies within the pretty pink grapefruit that rests on top of the fresh green lettuce. The other half? How simple and deliciously light this dish looks on a summer plate.

ingredients
1 Tablespoon extra-virgin olive oil
1 cup (about ½ large bunch) asparagus spears, ends removed
1 grapefruit, peeled and sectioned
2 cups chopped romaine lettuce
¼ cup shaved Parmesan cheese
Traditional Balsamic Vinaigrette (see page 64)

directions
Heat olive oil in a medium sauté pan. After asparagus ends have been removed, cut spears in half horizontally, then add to pan. Cook for 4–5 minutes, stirring occasionally. Add grapefruit sections and heat for an additional minute, then remove from heat.

Divide lettuce between two plates, topping each with equal parts asparagus, grapefruit, and Parmesan cheese. Divide balsamic vinegar dressing, drizzling evenly on top of each salad.

Want to make it vegan? Nix the Parmesan cheese and top with a vegan cheese substitute instead. You can also try adding nutritional yeast for a vegan cheese-like topping. Nutritional yeast is packed with nutrients, including vitamin B12, selenium, and folic acid. It's also salt-, sugar-, and gluten-free (check specific brands for certification). Find it in the bulk section at your health foods store or try Bragg's Premium Nutritional Yeast Seasoning (www.bragg.com).

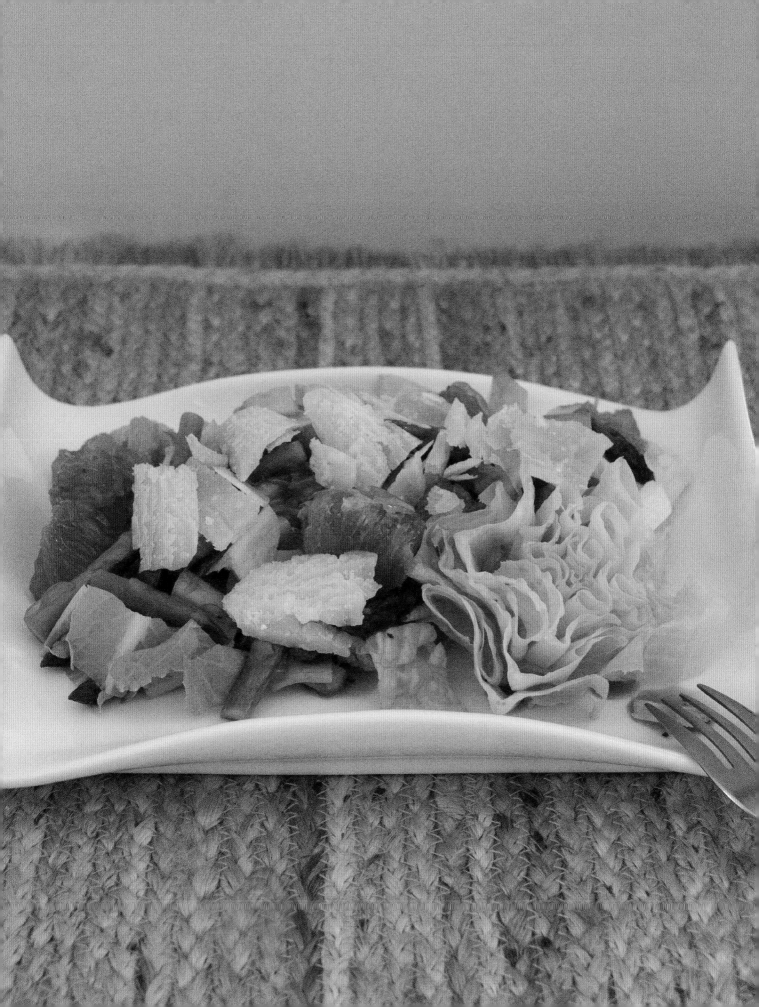

Black-Eyed Pea Quinoa Salad with Mint & Radishes

Makes 2–3 servings

This salad is a great substitute for ho-hum picnic dishes. Who wants the usual potato or macaroni salad when they can have this gorgeously fresh bite to eat instead?

ingredients
salad
1 cup cooked quinoa (red or white)
¾ cup cooked black-eyed peas
1 cup halved red and yellow cherry tomatoes
2 small red radishes, sliced
½ cup diced zucchini
2 fresh mint leaves, shredded
Honey Mustard Dressing (see page 62)

directions
Place all salad (quinoa through mint) ingredients into a large bowl and toss to combine.

Drizzle dressing over salad and toss again to combine. Keep chilled until ready to serve.

Want to make it vegan? Trade the honey in the dressing for agave or maple syrup.

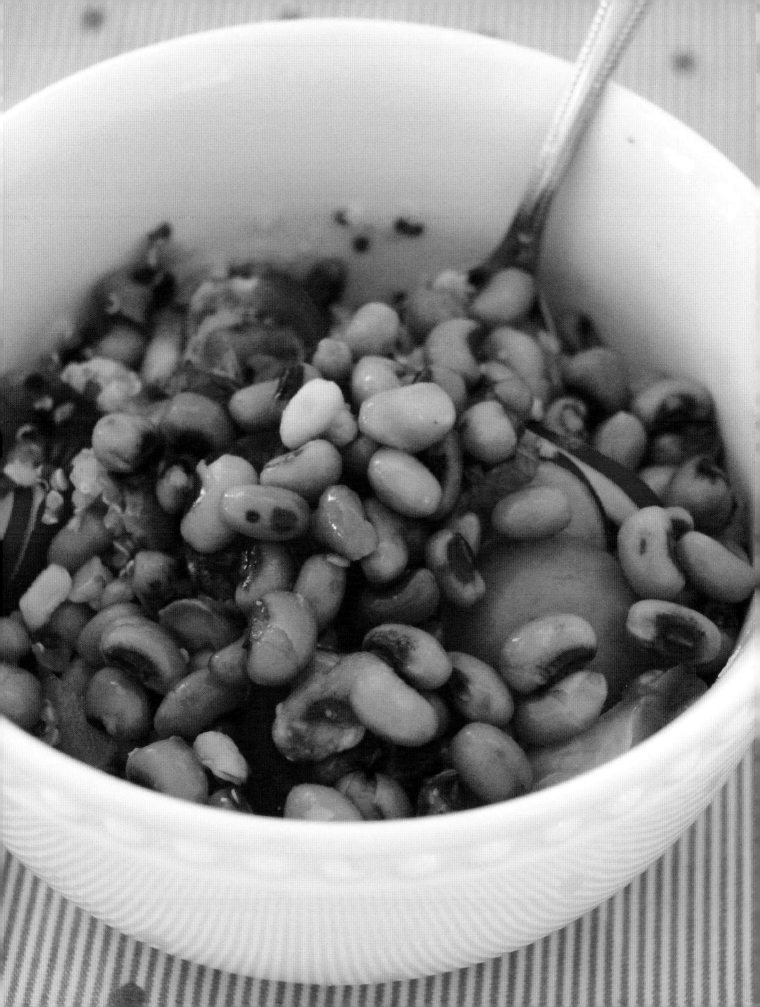

the main event

Spaghetti Squash Pasta
Parchment Paper–Steamed Salmon
Brown Butter & Thyme Pasta
Fiesta Quinoa Stir-Fry
Cheesy Tuna Tater Pie
Raw Zucchini Pasta
Raw Zucchini Pesto Noodles
Pineapple Goat Cheese Pizza
Honey Dijon Chickpea & Olive Pizza
Cauliflower Rice
Veggie Stuffed Peppers
Pimp Yo' Potato
Pineapple Sesame Tofu
Sloppy Faux Joes
Weeklong Veggie Chili
Mushroom Stroganoff
No-Fuss Burrito in a Bowl

It's dinner time! Here's the part where we decorate our plates with gorgeous veggies and herbs, gluten-free pasta, and even a few naughty dishes too, like pizza and cheesy potato pie. Hungry yet?

Spaghetti Squash Pasta

Makes approximately 2 cups

It is so much fun to watch this "pasta" spring to life! Bonus: It's simple enough to make that even kids will love lending a hand.

ingredients
1 spaghetti squash

directions
Preheat oven to 350°F. Cut the squash in half, lengthwise. Clean out the seeds and pulp before placing squash in a baking pan, cut-side up. Pour a cup of water in the pan and bake for about an hour, until the inside of squash is soft.

Allow 20 minutes for squash to cool, then, using a fork, scrape the squash from top to bottom. Continue this process until noodles begin to form.

Top noodles with your favorite sauce.

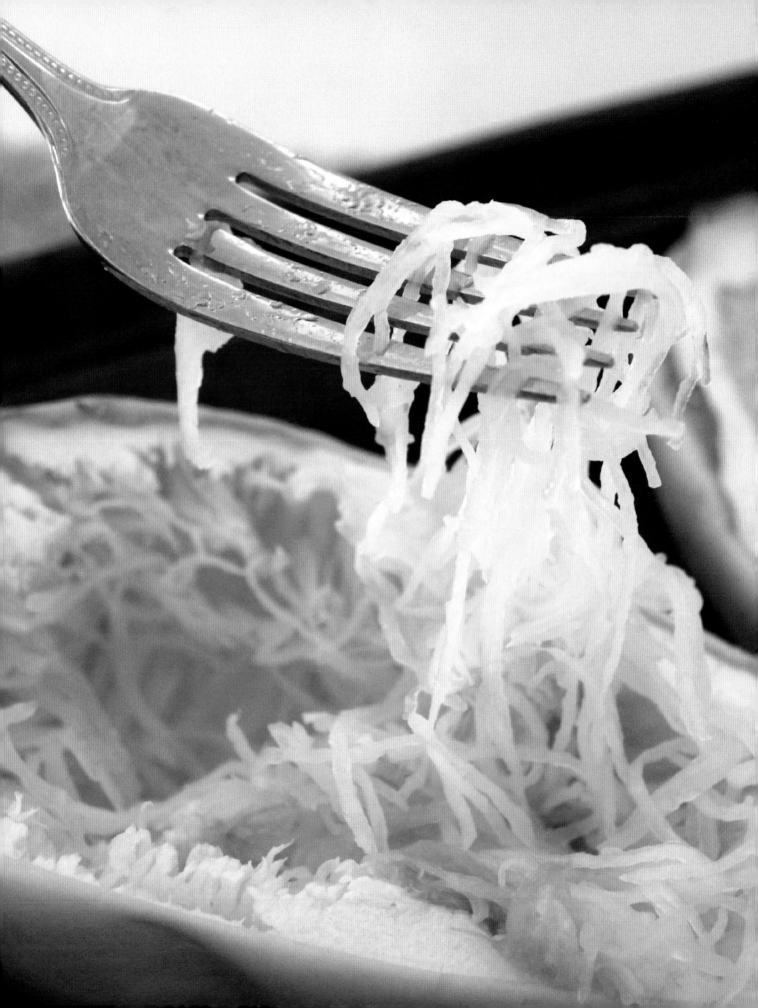

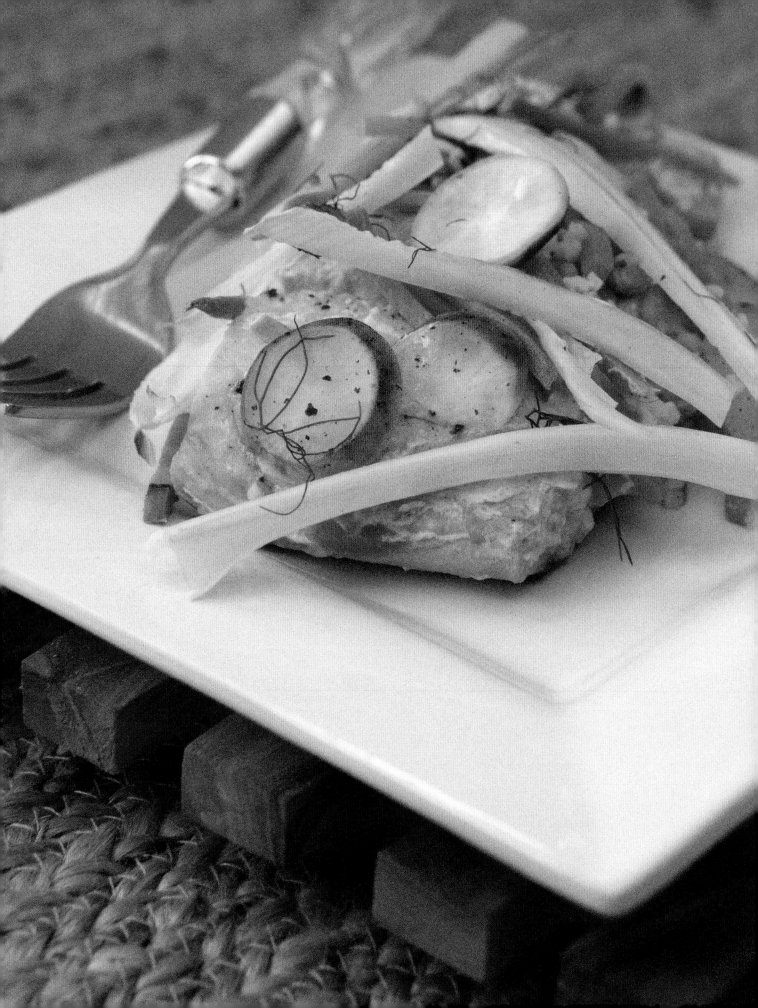

Parchment Paper–Steamed Salmon (vegan option)
Makes 1 serving

This recipe is the perfect option for a single guy or gal, or simply someone who is craving something simple and delicious for dinner. I have also made this dish the night before a busy day and packed it for an on-the-go meal. Serve on top of rice, quinoa, or spaghetti squash pasta (see page 104). It's also fabulous on its own!

ingredients
5- to 6-ounce salmon fillet
1 medium carrot, peeled and julienned or cut into matchsticks
½ fennel bulb, cut into matchsticks
2 red radish bulbs, thinly sliced
¼ small yellow onion, thinly sliced
juice of ¼ orange, seeds removed
2–3 garlic cloves, minced
sea salt and pepper to taste

directions
Preheat oven to 350°F. Prepare a sheet of parchment paper on a baking sheet.

Place salmon in center of baking sheet, then top with all ingredients. Bring right and left edges of parchment paper together in center, rolling to "crimp" the paper together. Do the same with each end, rolling until you have formed a parchment paper home for your fish.

Bake 25–30 minutes, depending on desired doneness.

Tip! No salmon? Try another fish you have on hand or trade it for extra-firm tofu to make the dish vegan.

Brown Butter & Thyme Pasta (vegan)

Makes 4 servings

This pasta is so visually refreshing—everything about it makes it feel like springtime has arrived at your table. I used Annie Chun's Pad Thai Rice Noodles in this dish for a lighter touch, but you can choose whatever pasta you like.

ingredients

8 ounces gluten-free pasta, prepared according to directions on package

2 medium zucchini, sliced thinly lengthwise (use regular or julienne peeler to make pasta ribbons)

2 Tablespoons vegan butter substitute

2 garlic cloves, minced

½ teaspoon sea salt

1 Tablespoon minced fresh thyme

ground pepper, to taste

directions

Place prepared pasta aside in a large bowl.

Melt butter in a medium saucepan over medium-high heat. Cook until the butter begins to brown, 2–3 minutes. Add garlic and zucchini, stirring often, until softened, about 3 minutes. Add sea salt, thyme, and pepper, stirring for an additional 1–2 minutes. Pour mixture over pasta, toss in bowl to coat and serve.

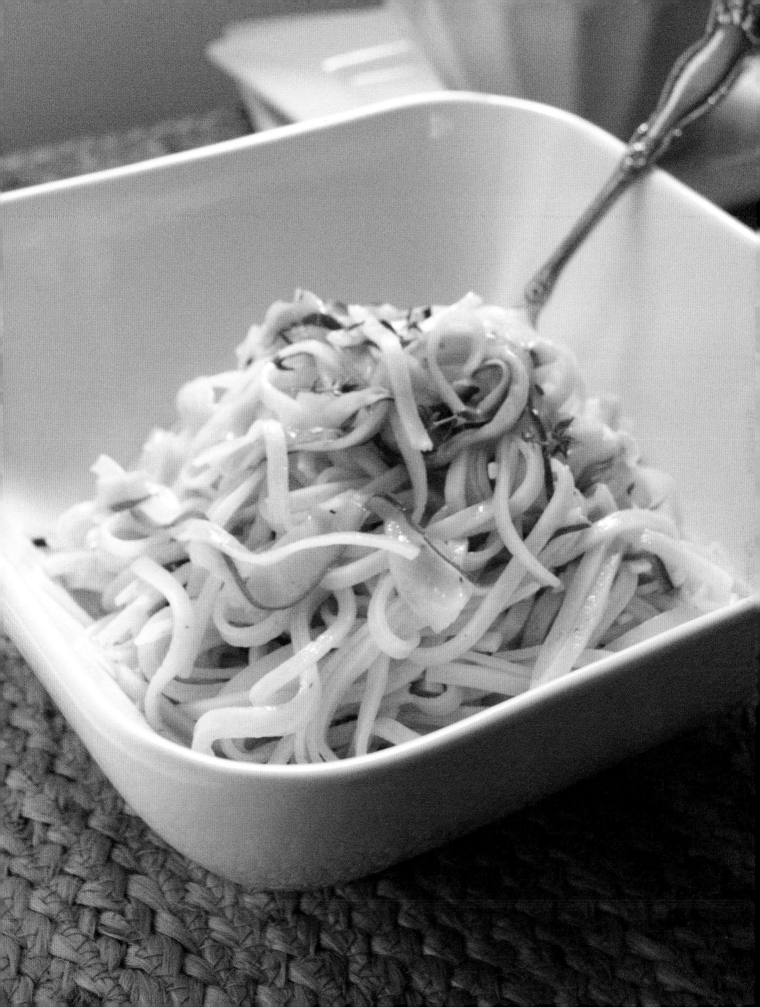

Fiesta Quinoa Stir-Fry (vegan option)

Makes 2 servings

Quinoa is a protein- and fiber-packed whole grain, giving it enough gusto to stand on its own in any dish. Top this stir-fry with sour cream, avocado, and lime for a festive and flavorful punch.

ingredients
2 Tablespoons extra-virgin olive oil
1 cup mixed bell peppers (red, yellow, orange, and green)
2 garlic cloves, minced
¼ cup chopped white onion
1 cup canned chickpeas
pinch of red chili pepper flakes
¼ teaspoon chili powder
1 cup cooked quinoa
1–2 lime wedges
regular or vegan sour cream, as desired
sliced avocado, as desired

directions
Heat olive oil in a sauté pan over medium heat. Add peppers, garlic, onion, chickpeas, red chili pepper flakes, and chili powder, stirring occasionally. After 3–4 minutes, add quinoa, continuing to cook for an additional 2–3 minutes.

Scoop into bowls and top with lime juice, sour cream, and avocado, as desired.

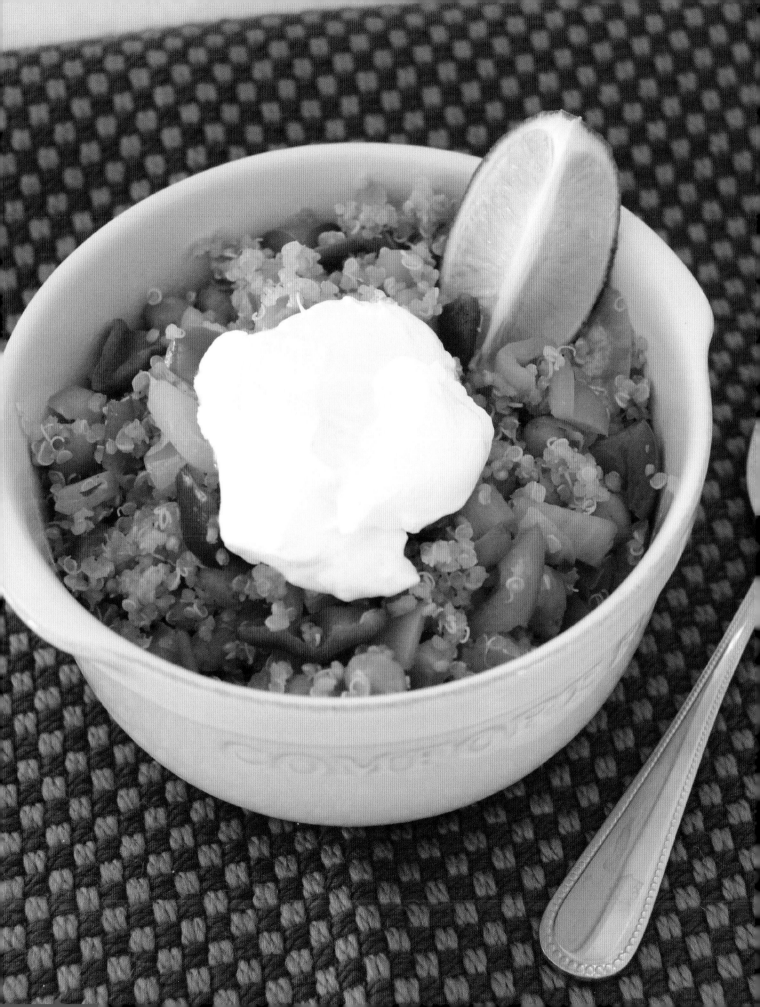

Cheesy Tuna Tater Pie (vegetarian option)

Serves 8

My mom used to make this for us as a special "treat" when we were growing up. When she recently found the recipe (originally from the side of a box of Hungry Jack® Instant Mashed Potatoes), I decided that it was necessary I find a way to make it gluten-free. The result? A slice of comfort food at its finest.

crust
1 cup Gluten-Free All-Purpose Baking Mix (see page 144)
½ cup gluten-free instant potato flakes
½ cup and 2 Tablespoons butter, cut into squares
4–5 Tablespoons water

caramelized onion
1 medium onion
¼ cup granulated sugar

filling
1 cup gluten-free cream of mushroom soup (try Progresso brand)
2 Tablespoons tapioca starch
¾ cup gluten-free instant potato flakes
1½ cups shredded cheddar cheese
1 5-ounce can albacore tuna in water
1 egg

directions

Preheat oven to 350°F. Begin caramelizing onion by following instructions on page 53. When finished, set aside until ready for use.

In a medium bowl, combine 1 cup flour with ½ cup potato flakes. Add squares of butter a few at a time to the mixture until all have been added. Use a fork or pastry blender to combine the mixture until it resembles a coarse mixture. Sprinkle mixture with water, 1 Tablespoon at a time, while tossing and mixing with fork.

Add water until dough is just moist enough to hold together. Press in bottom and up sides of ungreased 9- or 10-inch pan; flute edge. Reserve ½ onions for topping; sprinkle remaining onions over crust.

In a medium pot, combine mushroom soup and tapioca flour over low heat, whisking constantly until thoroughly combined. Remove from heat and set aside.

Add mushroom soup mixture to a medium bowl and combine with ¾ cup potato flakes, 1 cup of cheese, tuna, and egg, mixing well. Spoon mixture into a crust-lined pan. Bake for 25–30 minutes or until crust is golden brown.

Remove pie from oven (make sure to protect your hands!) and sprinkle with reserved ½ cup of onions and ½ cup of cheese. Bake an additional 5–10 minutes or until cheese is melted. Let stand for 5–10 minutes before slicing and serving.

Want to make it vegetarian? Nix the tuna and add ¼ teaspoon sea salt to the filling mixture.

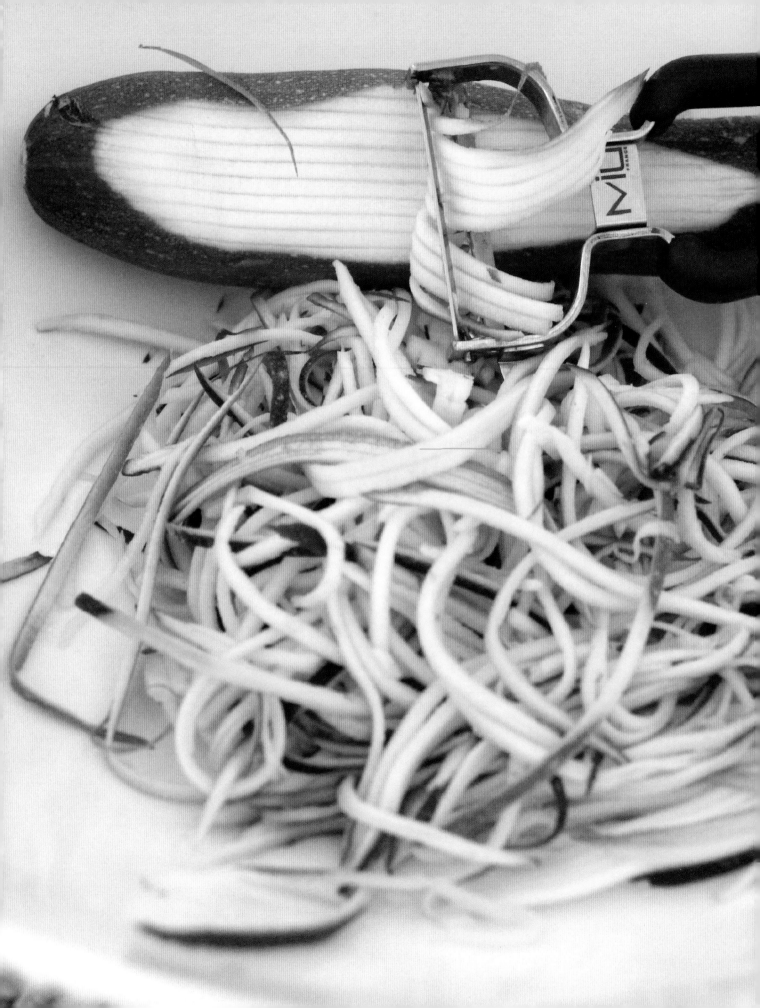

Raw Zucchini Pasta (vegan)

Makes 2½ to 3 cups

If simple kitchen wonders bring you joy, then you're about to love experimenting with a julienne peeler!

ingredients

2 medium organic zucchini

directions

Set zucchini on a cutting board and begin to pull julienne peeler lengthwise. Watch as "noodles" begin to form. Continue until all zucchini has been peeled.

Tip! Serve raw or lightly steam with other veggies for a tasty pasta dish.

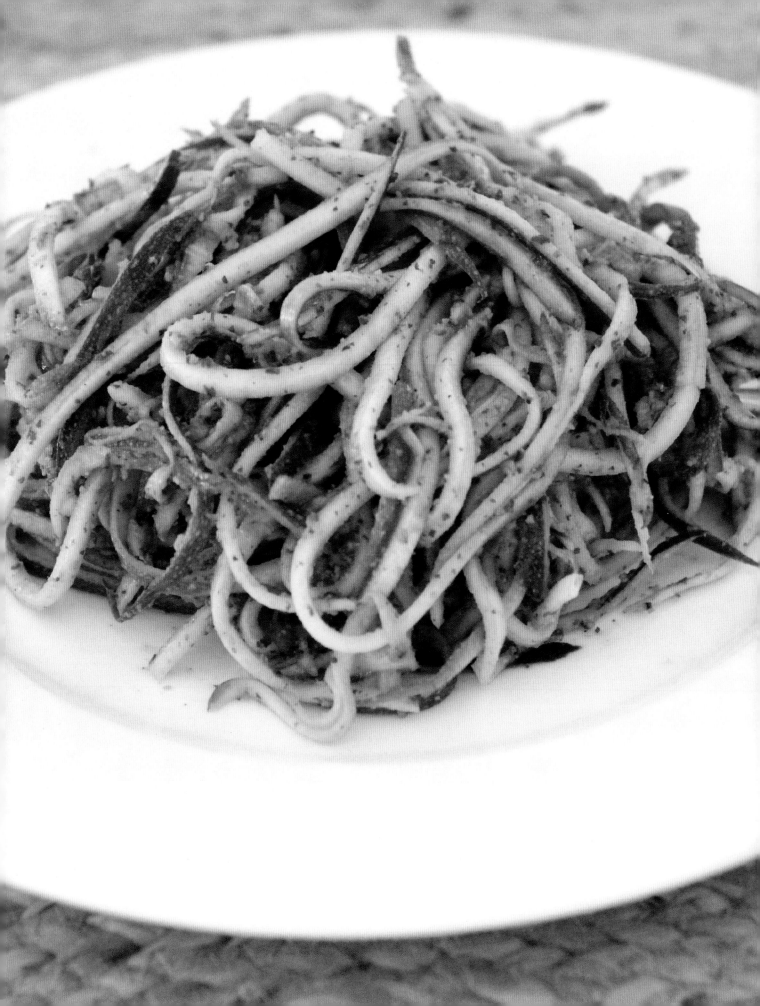

Raw Zucchini Pesto Noodles

Makes two 1-cup servings

This dish is what happens when the zucchini "pasta" on page 115 and the Roasted Walnut Herb Pesto on page 68 get together and make food magic. Serve these noodles next to grilled fish or roasted veggies for a well-rounded dish. They also stand wonderfully on their own. Top with goat cheese for an extra kick or vegan mozzarella if you are seeking a non-dairy meal.

2 cups raw zucchini pasta
2 Tablespoons Roasted Walnut Herb Pesto
regular or vegan cheese, if desired

In a medium bowl, combine zucchini pasta and pesto, stirring until combined. Top with cheese, if desired, and serve.

Tip! This makes for a delicious side dish when served with the Parchment Paper Salmon on page 106.

Pineapple Goat Cheese Pizza with Roasted Walnut Herb Pesto (vegan option)

Makes 4 pizza slices

ingredients

1 8-inch gluten-free pizza crust
½ cup Roasted Walnut Herb Pesto (see page 68)
1 cup pineapple, diced
½ cup sliced grape or cherry tomatoes
2 ounces goat cheese, crumbled
¼ cup chopped green onions
½ cup fresh arugula leaves

directions

Preheat oven according to pizza crust instructions. Prepare pizza crust accordingly, then top with Roasted Walnut Herb Pesto, pineapple, tomatoes, goat cheese, and green onions. Bake pizza according to package instructions. Remove pizza from oven and top with fresh arugula. Slice and serve.

Want to make it vegan? Use a vegan pizza crust and swap the goat cheese for your vegan cheese of choice.

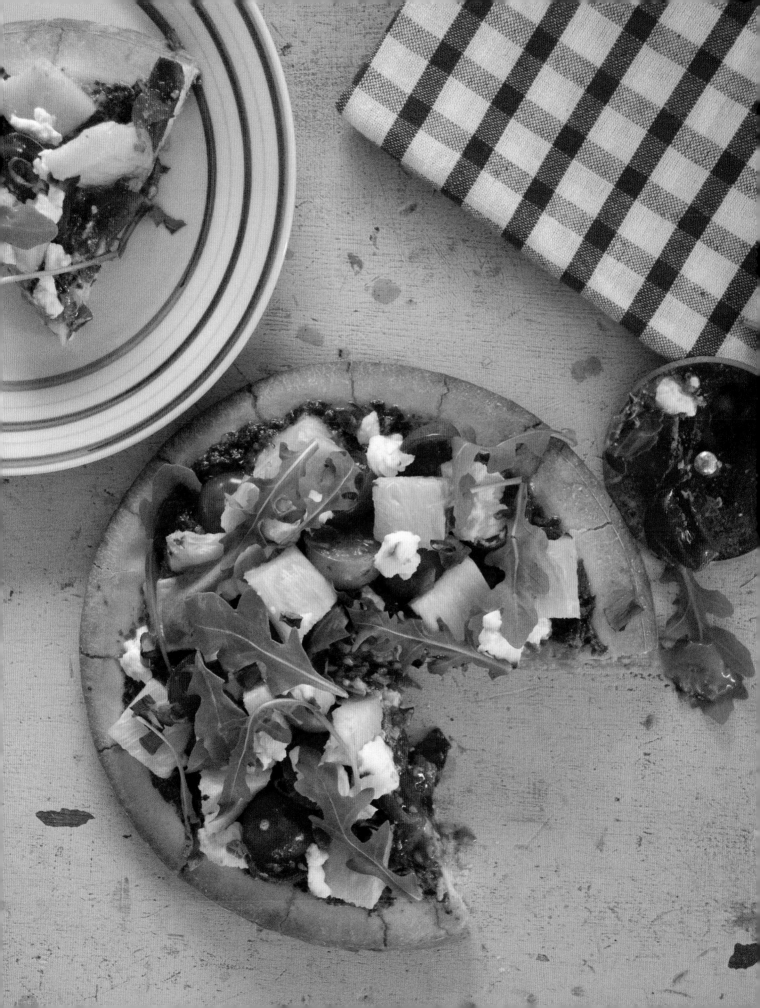

Honey Dijon Chickpea & Olive Pizza with Feta Cheese and Grapes

Makes 4 pizza slices

Prior to going gluten-free, one of my favorite pizzas was a honey dijon and feta cheese combination served on a pita "pizza" from a local Lebanese restaurant. This gluten-free version is my ode to that very pizza!

ingredients

1 8-inch gluten-free pizza crust
2 Tablespoons goat cheese, crumbled
½ cup red seedless grapes, cut lengthwise
¼ cup cooked chickpeas
¼ cup pitted and chopped Kalamata olives
¼ cup feta cheese, crumbled
1 Tablespoon pine nuts
1 Tablespoon minced green onions
1½ Tablespoons Honey Mustard Dressing (see page 62)

directions

Preheat oven according to pizza crust instructions. Prepare pizza crust accordingly, then top with goat cheese, grapes, chickpeas, olives and feta cheese. Sprinkle pine nuts and green onions on top.

Bake pizza according to package instructions.

Remove pizza from oven and drizzle with Honey Mustard Dressing. Slice and serve.

Want to make your own pizza crust? Check out this recipe for homemade gluten-free dough: http://sincerelycaroline.com/recipe/pizza-crust/

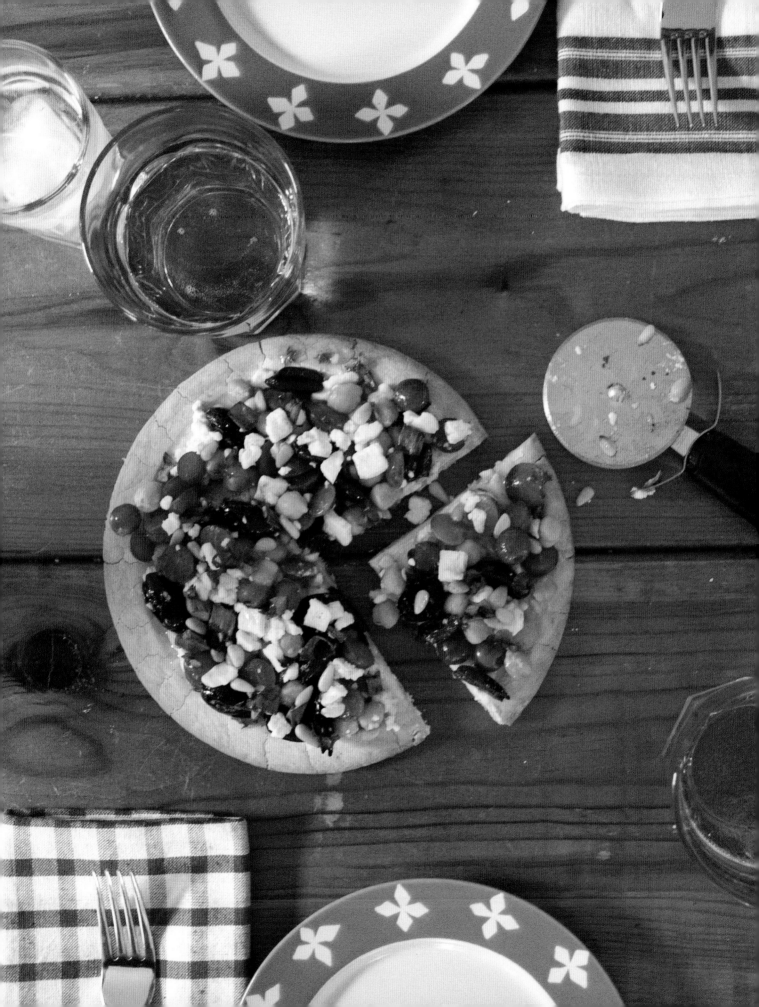

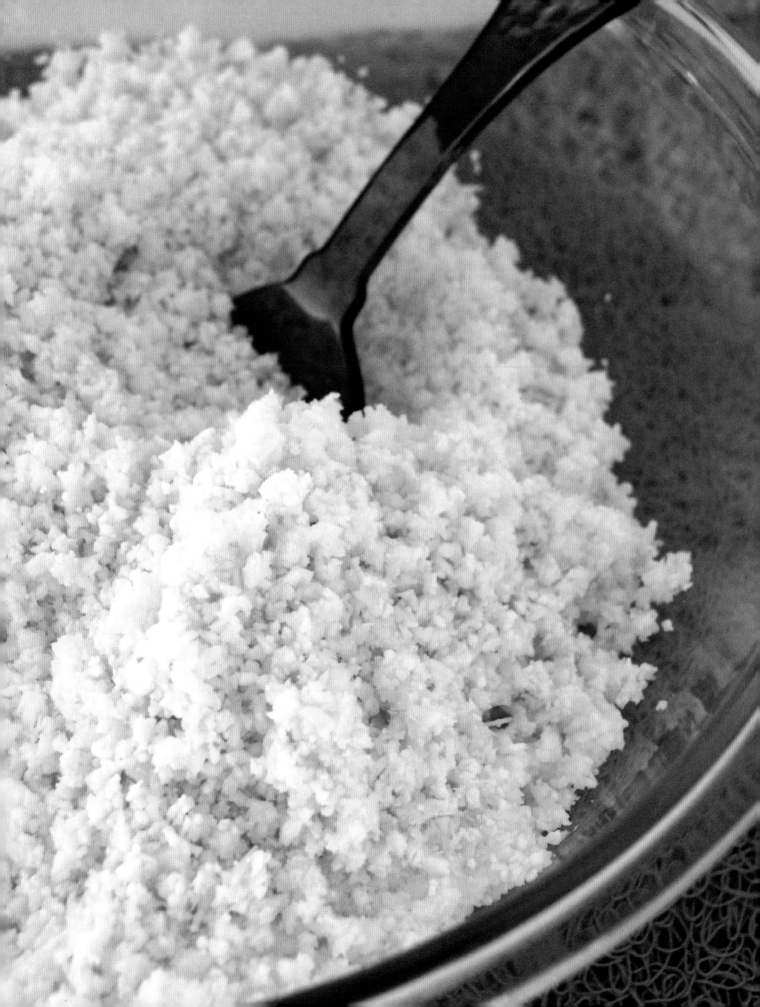

Cauliflower Rice
Makes 4–5 cups, depending on size of cauliflower

Sure, rice is yummy, but sometimes it's fun to shake things up. Try this veggie option in some of your favorite rice or pasta dishes for a new spin.

ingredients
1 head of fresh cauliflower

directions
Chop cauliflower into chunks, then place into a food processor. Pulse until a rice-like texture begins to form. Store in an airtight container in the refrigerator until ready for use.

Veggie Stuffed Peppers (vegan option)

Makes 4 servings

You won't miss the usual ground meat and rice with these filled-to-the-brim delights! By adding lentils and cauliflower rice to this traditional recipe, you'll discover a filling vegetarian dinner option.

ingredients
4 medium bell peppers (any color)
2 Tablespoons extra-virgin olive oil
⅔ cup cooked or canned lentils
1½ cups cauliflower rice (see page 123)
½ cup diced celery (about 2 medium stalks)
1 cup yellow onion, diced
2 garlic cloves, minced
2 Tablespoons minced fresh oregano
1 Tablespoon minced fresh thyme
2 ounces goat cheese, crumbled
1 14.5-ounce can of diced tomatoes
½ teaspoon sea salt
¼ teaspoon garam masala spice
ground pepper, as desired
½ cup tomato sauce
⅓ cup shredded Parmesan cheese

directions
Preheat oven to 350°F. Remove core and excess seeds from each of the peppers. Place peppers, standing up, in a shallow 8×8-inch baking dish. Set dish aside.

In a medium pan, heat about 2 Tablespoons of olive oil over medium heat. Add lentils, cauliflower rice, celery, onion, and garlic, sautéing for 6–7 minutes, until vegetables soften. Remove vegetables from heat and drain excess liquid from mixture if necessary. Set aside.

In a medium bowl, combine oregano, thyme, goat cheese, diced tomatoes, sea salt, garam masala, and ground pepper. Stir together, then slowly add reserved vegetable mixture. Mix thoroughly until combined.

Using a spoon, stuff each pepper with the vegetable mixture, making sure to pack in the ingredients until top is overflowing. Top each pepper with Parmesan cheese and then place tomato sauce in the bottom of the dish, around the peppers.

Bake for 25–30 minutes, until cheese begins to brown.

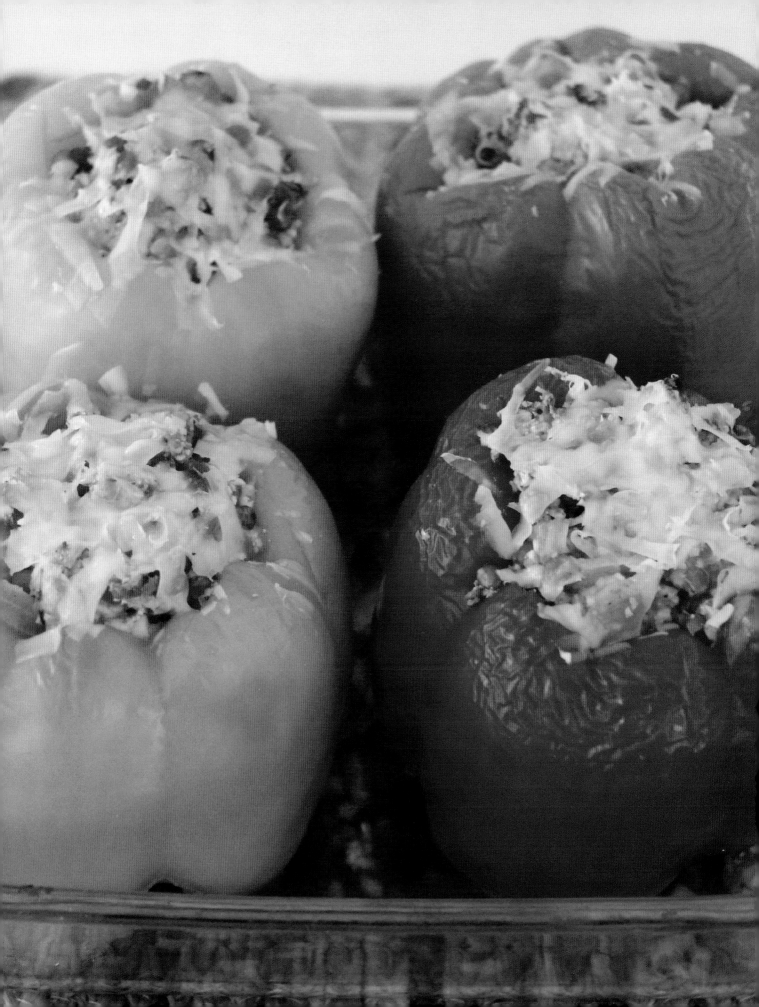

Pimp Yo' Potato (vegan options)

It's no secret that one of the best ways to this Irish girl's heart is through her potatoes. I love 'em baked, mashed, stuffed, and even fried. Here, I offer up a few suggestions for a new take on the timeless baked potato. Do you notice that I didn't include measurements? That's because you are supposed to stuff them as you please. The more ingredients that topple over the sides, the better!

NOTE: All potatoes are best when brushed with olive oil, sprinkled with salt and placed on a baking sheet in the oven for 40–55 minutes (depending on potato size).

Fiesta Potato
Heat olive oil in a sauté pan, then add a variety of mixed peppers, onion, chili powder, black beans, and corn. Heat for 5–6 minutes, stirring occasionally. Stuff into a baked russet potato and top with lime juice, sour cream, salsa, and fresh avocado.

Greek Potato
Stuff a baked sweet potato with canned artichokes, feta cheese, pitted black and green olives, and toasted pine nuts.

Thai-Style Potato
In a medium bowl, mix together about ¼ cup of sour cream and 1 teaspoon red curry paste, then set aside. Stuff a russet potato with canned chickpeas (rinsed and drained), sour cream mixture, minced fresh ginger, and toasted unsweetened shredded coconut.

Health Nut Potato
Heat olive oil in a sauté pan, then add fresh kale, chopped yellow squash, minced garlic, precooked or canned lentils, and cooked quinoa. Cook for 5–6 minutes, stirring occasionally. Stuff kale mixture into a baked sweet potato and top with nutritional yeast, sea salt, and ground pepper as desired.

Did you know? Not only does nutritional yeast give dishes a wonderful cheesy flavor, but it also offers 6 grams of protein per 2 Tablespoons. See page 98 for more details.

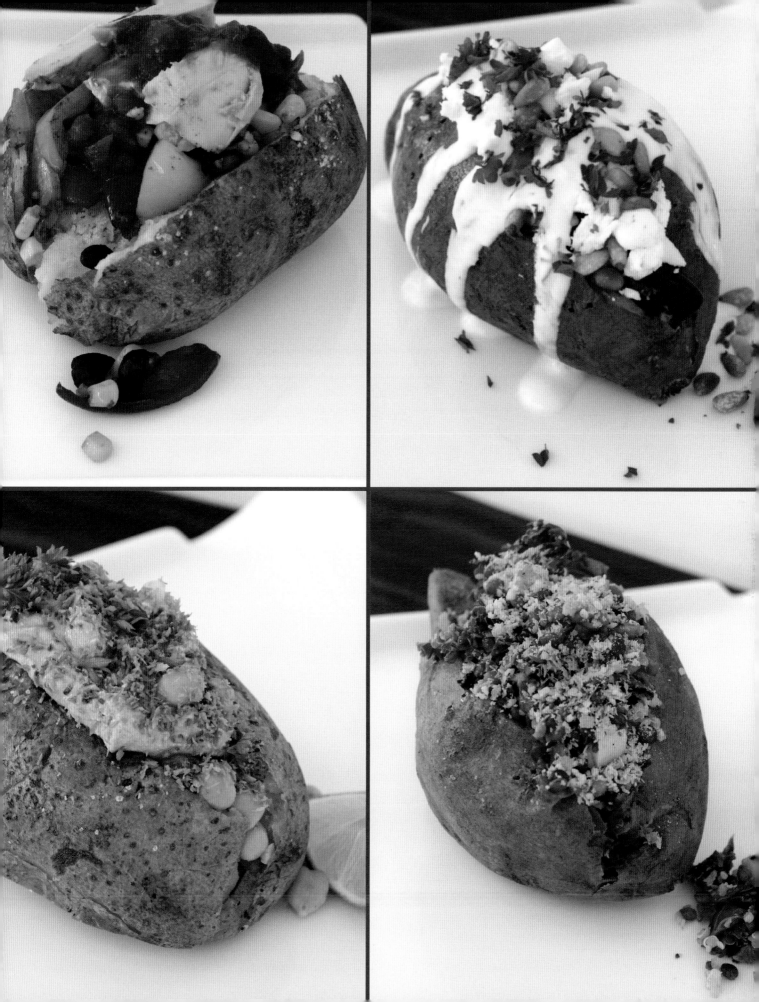

Pineapple Sesame Tofu (vegan option)
Makes 2 servings

It might sound like a strange pairing, but this dish is seriously OMG-delicious. Serve it over prepared brown rice or quinoa for a filling dinner. Oh, and the leftovers make for a stellar lunch the next day.

ingredients
3 Tablespoons tamari
¼ cup water
1 teaspoon mirin rice cooking wine
¼ teaspoon crushed red pepper
3 Tablespoons honey or maple syrup
1 Tablespoon minced garlic
1 Tablespoon minced ginger
1 teaspoon cornstarch
1 Tablespoon extra-virgin olive oil
½ block of extra firm tofu, cubed
1½ cups cubed fresh pineapple
½ cup chopped green onions, cut into 1-inch pieces

directions
Combine tamari, water, mirin, red pepper, honey, garlic, ginger, and cornstarch in a medium bowl, whisking together. Toss tofu cubes in the marinade and set aside, allowing it to sit for at least 15 minutes.

Prepare skillet by heating olive oil over high heat. When oil becomes hot, add pineapple, stirring occasionally for 2–3 minutes. Add marinated tofu, leaving as much sauce in the bowl as possible, and sauté for 1–2 minutes. Add half of the remaining marinade to the skillet. Let sauce reduce and thicken, stirring occasionally for 1–2 minutes, then remove from heat. Stir in green onions.

Serve over brown rice or quinoa.

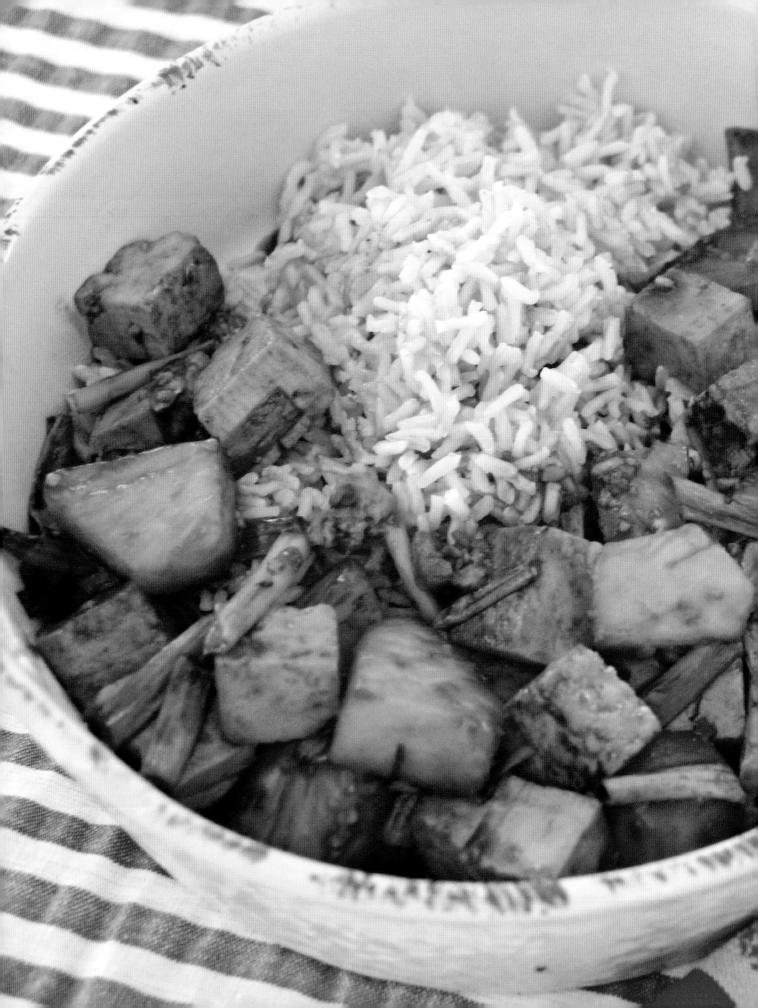

Sloppy Faux Joes (vegan option)

Makes 6–8 servings (depending on bun size)

You won't miss the meat in this veggie spin on the old, wonderfully messy classic!

ingredients

29 ounces tomato sauce
3 garlic cloves, minced
½ teaspoon ground mustard
½ teaspoon dried oregano
1 teaspoon chili powder
¼ teaspoon red chili pepper flakes
½ teaspoon sea salt
3 Tablespoons honey or agave syrup
2 Tablespoons olive oil
½ medium yellow onion, diced
½ cup diced red pepper
½ cup diced green pepper
1 cup diced eggplant
1 cup diced mushrooms
gluten-free sandwich buns
regular or vegan shredded cheese, if desired (for topping)

directions

In a medium pot, combine tomato sauce, garlic, ground mustard, oregano, chili powder, red chili pepper flakes, sea salt, and honey, stirring until combined. Simmer with lid on over low heat for 10 minutes.

In a medium sauté pan, combine olive oil, onion, red pepper, green pepper, eggplant, and mushrooms, stirring throughout and cooking over medium heat for 6–8 minutes, until vegetables are tender. Remove from heat and add to sauce mixture, stirring until combined. Simmer for an additional 8–10 minutes.

Toast the gluten-free buns for 5–6 minutes before topping with Sloppy Faux mixture. Scoop out with a slotted spoon to avoid excess juice that may cause bread to become mushy. Top with shredded cheese (if desired) and serve.

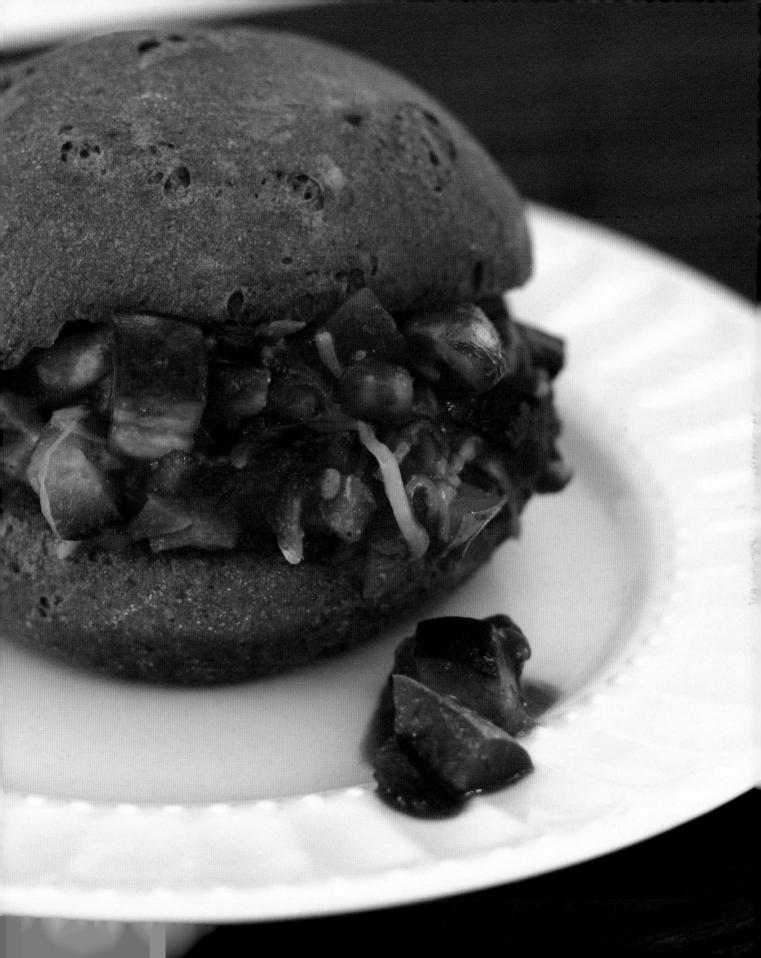

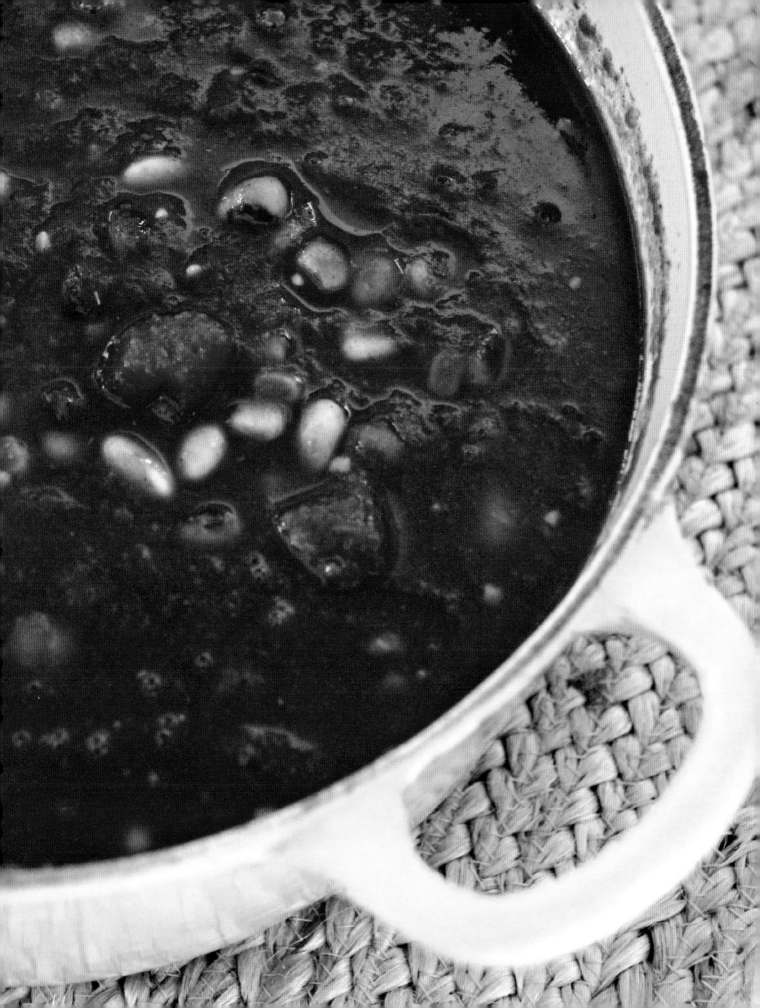

Weeklong Veggie Chili
Makes 10–12 servings

This is one of my favorite dishes to make at the start of a week. Dan and I pour it over whole grain brown rice or quinoa on the first night (topped with avocado, sour cream, and cheese, of course!), then have the rest for leftovers. If we get tired of it midweek, then we put it in a resealable container and pop it in the freezer. It's always good to have on hand when life gets busy!

ingredients
3 28-ounce cans tomato sauce
1 15.5-ounce can chickpeas, rinsed and drained
1 15.5-ounce can black beans, rinsed and drained
1 15.5-ounce can black-eyed peas, rinsed and drained
1 15.5-ounce can light red kidney beans, rinsed and drained
1 14.5-ounce can no-salt-added diced tomatoes
2 cups frozen corn
1½ cups frozen edamame
3 garlic cloves, minced
2 Tablespoons chili powder
1–2 teaspoons red pepper flakes
1 teaspoon sea salt

directions
Combine all ingredients in a large stock pot and simmer on low heat for at least an hour before serving. Stir occasionally throughout.

Mushroom Stroganoff (vegan option)

Makes 3 servings

ingredients

10 ounces gluten-free pasta, prepared according to package directions
4 teaspoons extra-virgin olive oil, divided
2 Tablespoons gluten-free flour
2 garlic cloves, minced
1 cup low-sodium vegetable broth
1 teaspoon tamari
1½ teaspoons Dijon mustard
½ cup low-fat regular or vegan sour cream
¼ teaspoon sea salt
ground pepper, as desired
½ yellow onion, diced
3 fresh sage leaves, minced
2 teaspoons minced fresh flat leaf parsley
4 ounces wild mushrooms, diced
2 large portabella mushroom caps, sliced

directions

Prepare gluten-free pasta according to package instructions and drain, then set aside.

Heat 2½ teaspoons of olive oil in a saucepan over medium heat. Whisk in flour and cook, stirring constantly, for about a minute. Add garlic and broth, continuing to whisk. Bring mixture to a simmer, then reduce the heat to low, whisking occasionally, for about 4 minutes.

While the broth mixture is cooking, measure tamari, Dijon mustard, sour cream, and sea salt in a small bowl. Stir to combine. When finished cooking, remove broth from heat and stir in tamari mixture. Top with ground pepper, as desired. Cover to keep warm and set aside.

Heat remaining 1½ teaspoons olive oil in a skillet. Add onion, cooking until tender, about 3 minutes. Add sage, parsley, wild mushrooms, and portabella mushrooms, cooking for 7–8 minutes. Stir in sauce that was set aside earlier.

Transfer gluten-free noodles to plates and top with mushroom mixture. Sprinkle with remaining 1 teaspoon of parsley and serve.

NOTE: Want a lighter dish? Serve Mushroom Stroganoff over Spaghetti Squash Pasta on page 104.

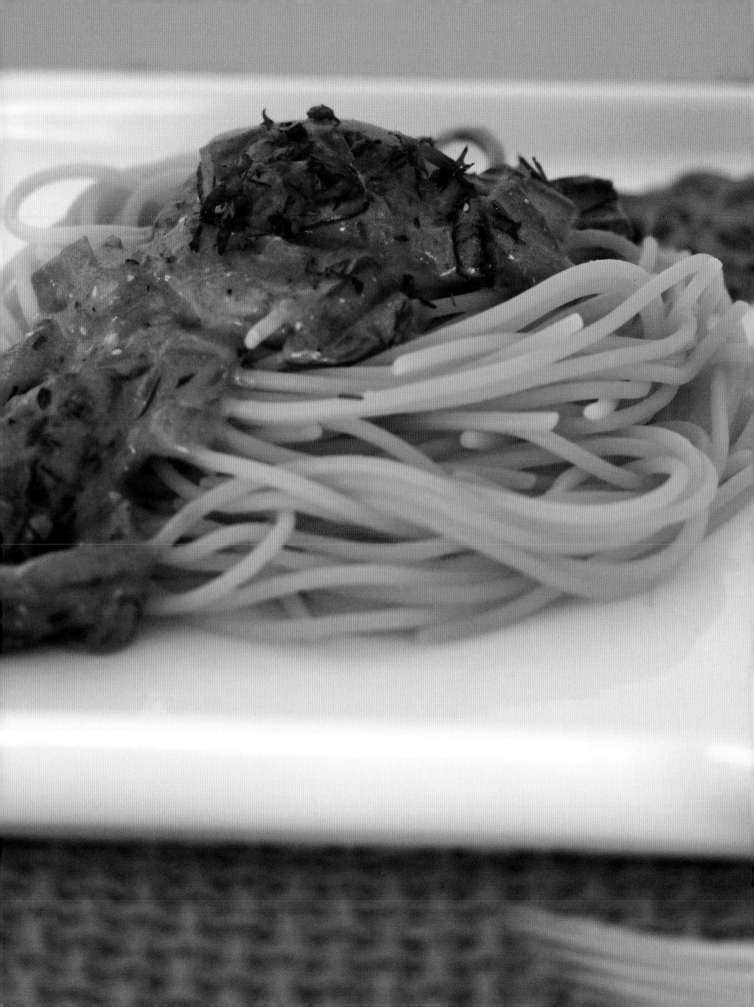

No-Fuss Burrito in a Bowl (vegan)

Makes 4 servings

ingredients

1 15-ounce can of black beans, drained and rinsed
1 15-ounce can of sweet corn, drained and rinsed
2 cups cooked brown rice
1 cup shredded cheddar cheese
1 cup shredded lettuce greens
1 avocado, sliced
½ cup vegan sour cream substitute
1 Tablespoon dairy-free milk
1 teaspoon chili powder
¼ teaspoon cumin
2 garlic cloves, minced
sea salt, to taste
1 lime

directions

Open and rinse black beans and sweet corn in a colander. Set aside.

Place ½ cup warm brown rice in a bowl and top with ¼ cup shredded cheese to allow it to melt. Top with ½ cup black beans and corn mixture, then ¼ cup shredded lettuce. Slice ¼ avocado and place on top.

Prepare dressing by whisking together sour cream, dairy-free milk, chili powder, cumin, garlic, and salt. Drizzle ¼ dressing mixture on top of burrito bowl. Squeeze the juice of ¼ fresh lime on top to finish preparation.

Repeat above steps three more times for a total of four servings.

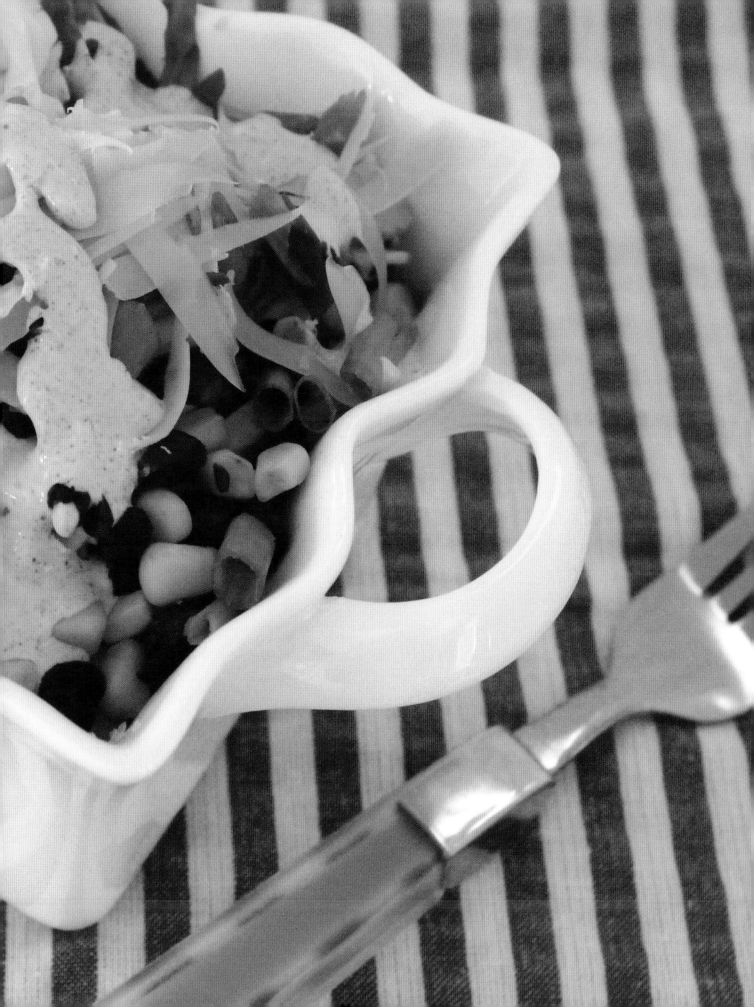

something sweet

Pistachio-Crusted Orange and Dark Chocolate Cookies
Frozen Chocolate Banana Peanut Bites
Gluten-Free All-Purpose Baking Mix
Oatmeal Crust
Chocolate Mint Dessert Smoothie
Apple Cheesecake Pie
Peanut Butter Protein Fudge
Classic Oatmeal Raisin Cookies
Nuts-About-Chocolate Clusters
Sunflower Butter & Jelly Cookies
Peanut Butter & Banana Cupcakes

There's no doubt about it: I have a serious sweet tooth. In fact, it's for that very reason that a large portion of my philosophy came into fruition. I have tried nixing sugar completely and it's just not something that works for me. It's my belief that if we allow small exceptions along the way, then it will keep us from gorging on an entire cake later.

I have definitely learned how to keep my portions in check, but I can honestly say that I have something sweet almost every day. It might only be a small square of chocolate or glass of chocolate almond milk, but it's enough to keep this gal happy.

Pistachio Crusted Orange and Dark Chocolate Cookies
Makes 24 cookies

ingredients
1 flaxseed egg (1 Tablespoon flaxseed meal, plus 3 Tablespoons warm water)
1 cup coconut sugar
zest and juice of 1 medium orange
1 cup vegan butter substitute
1½ cups almond meal
1 cup white rice flour
¼ teaspoon salt
1 teaspoon baking powder
1 cup vegan chocolate chips
¼ cup unsweetened dairy-free milk (almond, coconut, hemp, etc.)
⅓ cup unsalted pistachios, chopped

directions
Preheat oven to 350°F. Prepare two baking sheets by lining with parchment paper or baking mats. Set aside.

Combine flaxseed meal and warm water in a small bowl, then set aside.

Measure coconut sugar, orange zest and juice, and vegan butter into a medium bowl. Using a hand or standing mixer on medium speed, combine ingredients. Add in flaxseed mixture, almond meal, white rice flour, sea salt, and baking powder, mixing again on medium speed until ingredients are just combined. Do not over-mix or dough will become tough.

Drop cookie dough by rounded Tablespoonfuls onto prepared baking sheet. Freeze for 5 minutes. After removing from freezer, press center of each cookie with thumb, then immediately place tray into oven. Bake 18–20 minutes, until golden brown.

While cookies are baking, measure chocolate chips and dairy-free milk into a small pot. Place over low heat, whisking constantly until mixture becomes smooth. Immediately remove from heat to avoid burning.

After cookies have been removed from oven, drizzle chocolate on top of each, then sprinkle with crushed pistachios. Freeze to solidify chocolate before serving.

NOTE: Don't have coconut sugar? Use granulated sugar for equally yummy cookies!

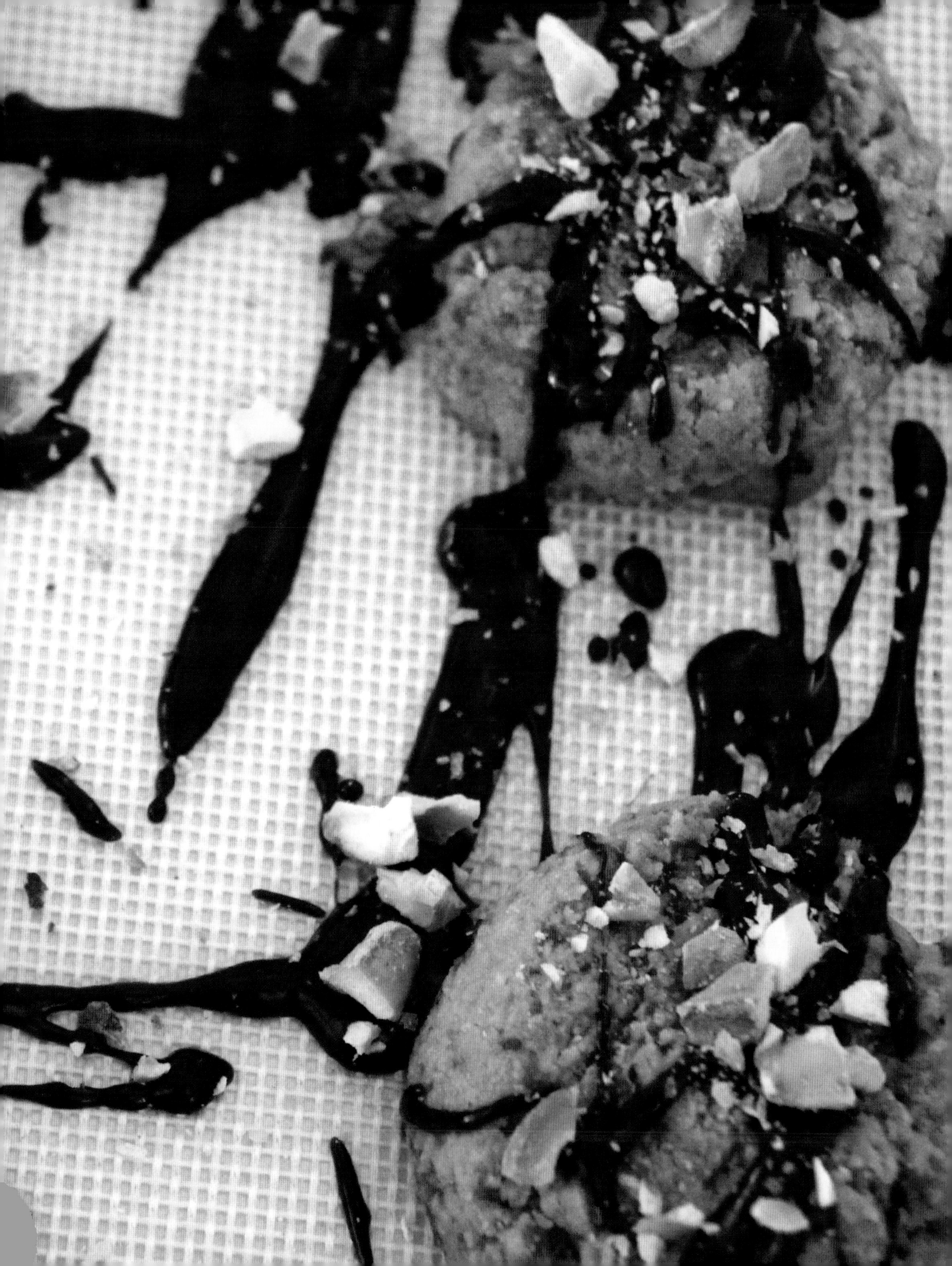

Frozen Chocolate Banana Peanut Bites

Makes 24–26 bites

When we were younger, my sister was 100 percent obsessed with those banana and chocolate popsicles you could buy from the ice cream man. I thought she was *Eeeew, gross!* and stuck with my chocolate fudgesicle instead. These days, I've gotten over my fear of bananas and I love to make these bites for a quick treat. The lil' sister loves them too!

ingredients
2 ripe bananas
2 cups vegan chocolate chips
½ cup dairy-free milk (almond, coconut, hemp, etc.)
½ cup unsalted peanuts, crushed

directions
Prepare a large baking sheet by lining it with parchment paper or baking mat. Set aside.

Slice each banana into ½-inch thick circles, then set aside.

In a small saucepan, melt chocolate and milk over low heat, stirring constantly until smooth. Remove from heat.

Drop banana slices into the chocolate four to five at a time, then remove from chocolate using a slotted spoon. Hold each banana over top of chocolate allowing excess to drip off before placing it onto the baking sheet. Repeat this process until all bananas are covered in chocolate. Sprinkle the chocolate covered banana slices with peanuts, then place tray in freezer for at least one hour, until chocolate has hardened.

Transfer frozen slices to a resealable container and place back in freezer until ready to serve.

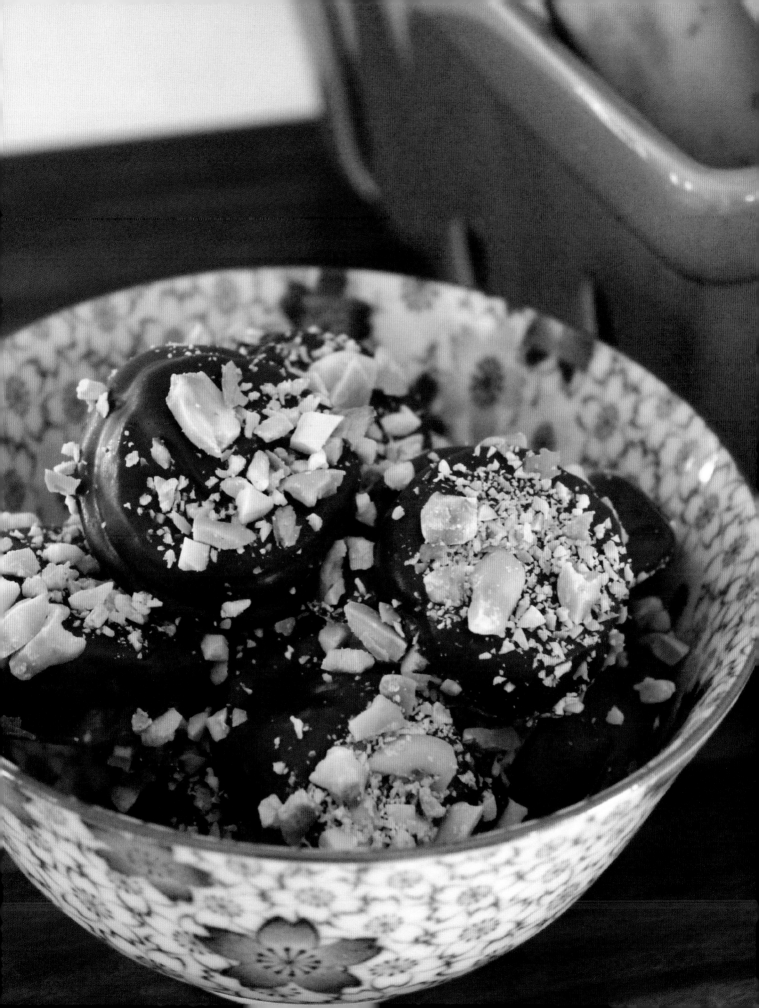

Gluten-Free All-Purpose Baking Mix

ingredients
¾ cup almond meal/flour
1 cup brown rice flour
¾ cup tapioca flour
½ cup arrowroot starch

directions
Mix flours in a medium bowl until thoroughly combined.

Oatmeal Crust

Makes 1 crust

I made this oatmeal crust its own recipe because it can be used for a number of other recipes including pies, breakfast recipes (see page 39), and dessert.

ingredients
½ cup and 2 Tablespoons vegan butter substitute, melted
½ cup brown sugar
1 cup Gluten-Free All-Purpose Baking Mix (see page 144)
1 cup gluten-free old-fashioned rolled oats

directions
In a medium bowl, combine all ingredients, breaking up brown sugar lumps by pressing against the sides of bowl with a fork. Set aside until ready for use.

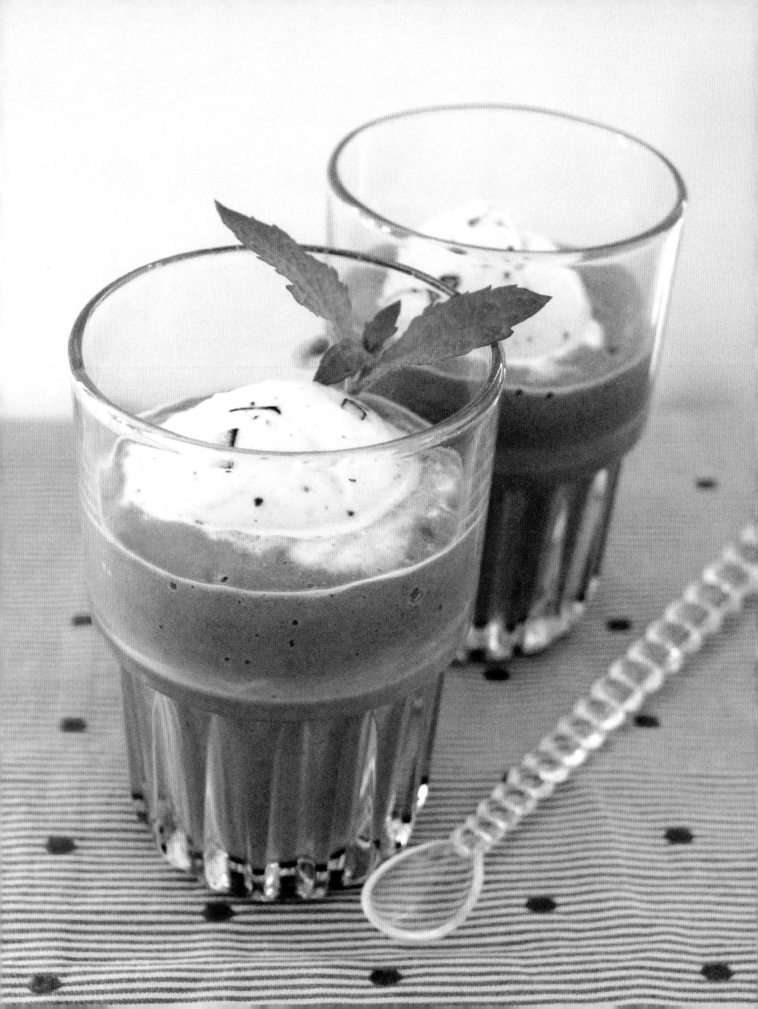

Chocolate Mint Dessert Smoothie (vegan)

Makes 2 servings

Talk about a balanced smoothie! Healthy ingredients with a smidge of something naughty make this drink a perfect after-dinner treat.

ingredients
½ Bartlett, Bosc or Anjou pear
½ avocado, peeled and pitted
⅓ cup dairy-free milk (almond, coconut, hemp, etc.)
½ Tablespoon raw cacao powder
1 fresh mint leaf
2 small scoops of dairy-free mint chocolate chip ice cream (optional)

directions
Blend pear, avocado, milk, cacao powder, and mint in a high-speed blender. Divide mixture between two glasses and top each with a scoop of ice cream, if desired.

Apple Cheesecake Pie with Oatmeal Crust (vegan)

Makes 12 servings

ingredients

1 prepared oatmeal crust (see page 145)
2 Tablespoons vegan butter substitute
¼ cup brown sugar
½ teaspoon cinnamon
1 medium apple, cut into slices
8 ounces vegan cream cheese substitute
12 ounces firm silken tofu
⅔ cup pure maple syrup
1 Tablespoon pure vanilla extract

directions

Preheat oven to 350°F. Press prepared oatmeal crust into an 8-inch pie pan until evenly distributed. Set aside.

In a medium skillet, melt butter. Sprinkle brown sugar and cinnamon evenly throughout pan, then add apple slices. Cook over low-medium heat for 6–8 minutes, flipping slices halfway through cook time. Remove from heat. Line apple slices on bottom of prepared oatmeal crust, overlapping where necessary.

In a food processor, combine cream cheese, tofu, maple syrup, and vanilla, pulsing until smooth. Pour mixture into apple-lined oatmeal crust, then place cheesecake in oven, baking for 70 minutes, or until browned on top.

Allow cheesecake to cool in pan on a wire baking rack for 10 minutes before running a butter knife along the outside edges to loosen the crust. This will help keep the top of the cheesecake from cracking. Cheesecake should continue to cool on rack for an additional 30 minutes before placing in refrigerator to cool completely for at least 4 hours, or overnight.

How do you know when your cheesecake is done? The center of a cheesecake will always slightly wobble (until it fully sets), but a good test to make sure you won't end up with an uncooked cheesecake on your hands is to lightly tap the side of the pan with a spoon. If the entire top of the cheesecake moves, then you need to leave it in a bit longer. If you just see movement toward the center, then the cheesecake is done.

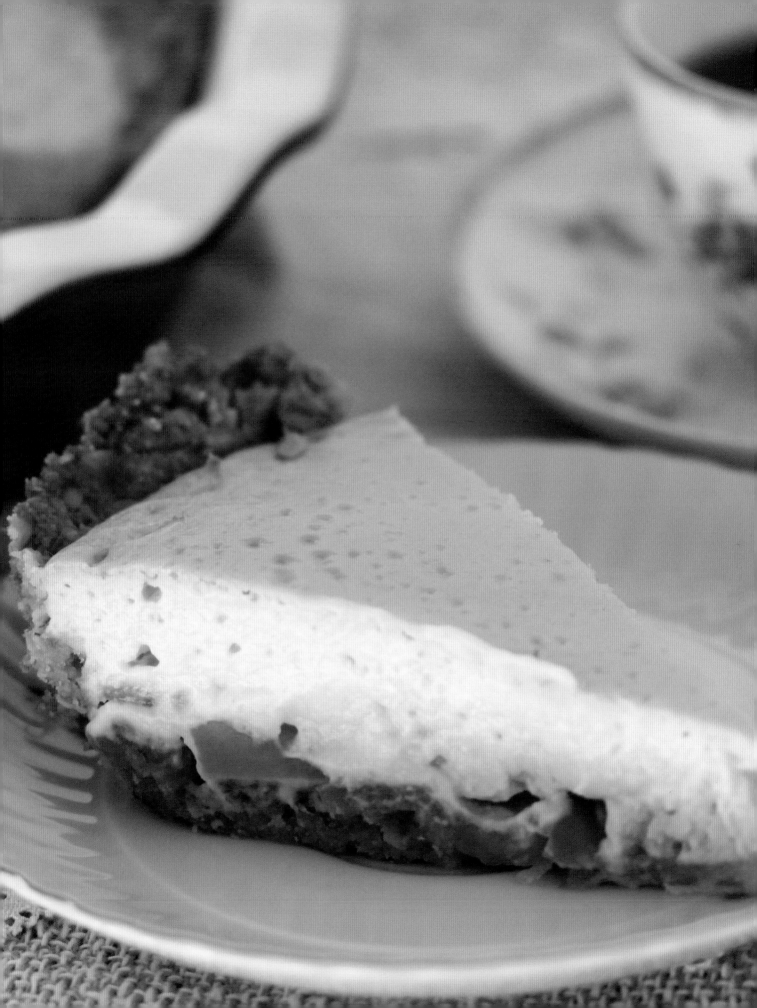

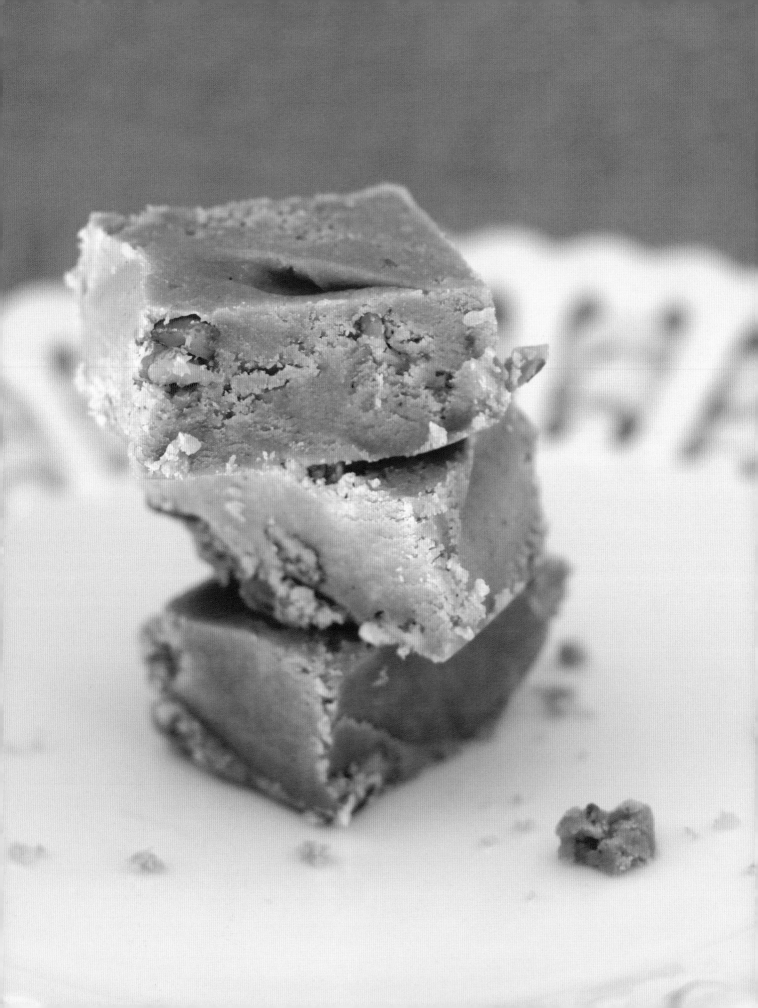

Peanut Butter Protein Fudge (vegan)

Makes approximately 25 fudge squares

ingredients

2½ cups powdered sugar
⅓ cup vegan protein powder
½ cup vegan butter substitute
1 cup light brown sugar
½ cup dairy-free milk (almond, coconut, hemp, etc.)
¾ cup natural peanut butter
1 teaspoon pure vanilla extract

directions

Add confectioners' sugar and protein powder to a large bowl, then set aside.

Melt butter in a medium saucepan over medium heat. Stir in brown sugar and milk. Bring to a boil and simmer for 2 minutes, stirring consistently. Remove from heat. Stir in peanut butter and vanilla. Pour over powdered sugar mixture, then beat until smooth. Pour into an 8x8-inch dish. Chill until firm, then cut into squares.

Classic Oatmeal Raisin Cookies (vegan)

Makes 18 cookies

ingredients

1 cup Gluten-Free All-Purpose Baking Mix (see page 144)
½ teaspoon baking soda
½ teaspoon baking powder
½ teaspoon sea salt
1 flaxseed egg (1 Tablespoon flaxseed meal plus 3 Tablespoons warm water)
½ cup vegan butter substitute, softened
⅓ cup sugar
½ cup light brown sugar, firmly packed
1 teaspoon pure vanilla extract
1½ cups gluten-free old-fashioned rolled oats
¾ cup raisins

directions

Preheat oven to 350°F. Prepare a baking sheet by lining with parchment paper or baking mat. Whisk together all dry ingredients; set aside.

Mix together flaxseed meal and water combination and set it aside.

Combine all wet ingredients with a hand mixer on low, increasing speed to high until color begins to lighten. Add in flaxseed mixture and continue to mix on medium until combined. Slowly stir the flour mixture into the creamed mixture until flour is fully incorporated. Fold in oats and raisins.

Scoop dough (about 2 Tablespoons per cookie) onto prepared pan, leaving about 2 inches between each cookie.

Bake 12–13 minutes, or until golden brown. Remove from oven, allowing cookies to sit on baking sheet for 5 minutes before transferring to a wire rack to cool completely.

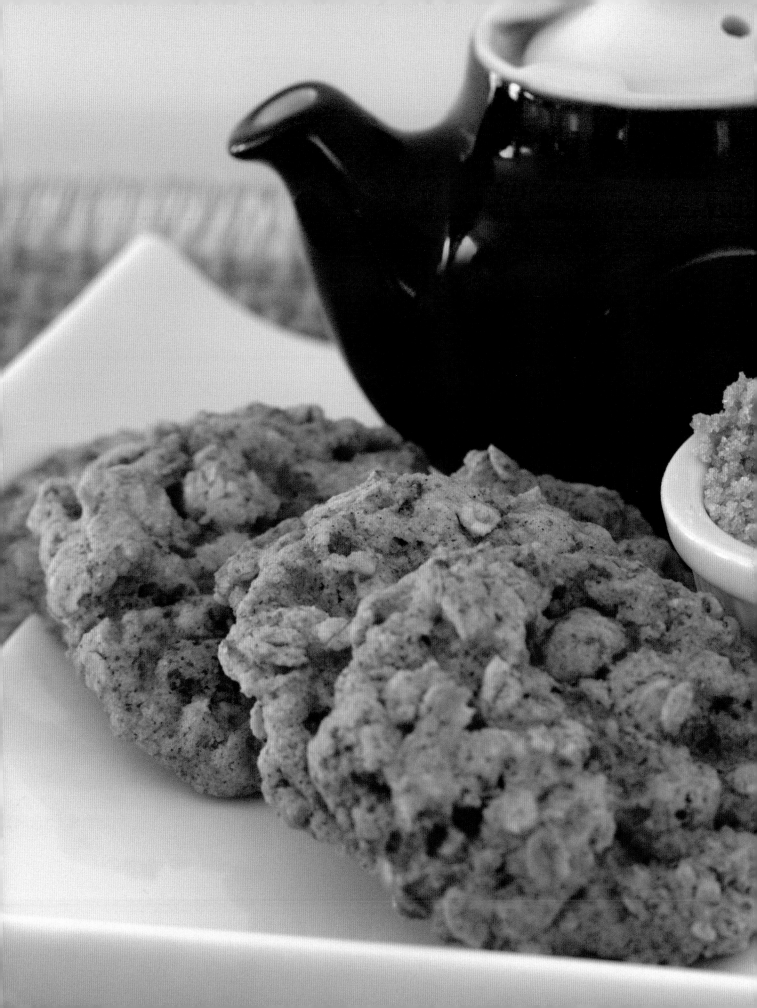

Nuts-About-Chocolate Clusters (vegan option)

Makes 24 clusters

ingredients

coconut oil, for brushing
½ cup raw, unsalted cashews
½ cup raw, unsalted walnuts
½ cup raw, unsalted almonds
½ cup raw, unsalted sunflower seeds
½ cup brown rice syrup
1 cup vegan or regular dark chocolate
¼ teaspoon sea salt

directions

Prepare two 12-cup mini muffin pans by brushing with coconut oil. Put aside.

Place cashews, walnuts, almonds, and sunflower seeds into a food processor and pulse until broken pieces remain.

Transfer nut mixture to a medium bowl and add brown rice syrup. Stir until well combined.

Add dark chocolate to a small pot, warming over medium heat. Stir constantly until smooth, then remove from heat.

Scoop approximately 1 rounded Tablespoon of mixture into each prepared muffin cup. Drizzle each nut cluster with dark chocolate. Place sea salt into palm of hand and sprinkle over each cluster.

Freeze nut clusters for 1 hour. Remove from cups by running a knife along the edges to loosen. Refrigerate in a container for storage.

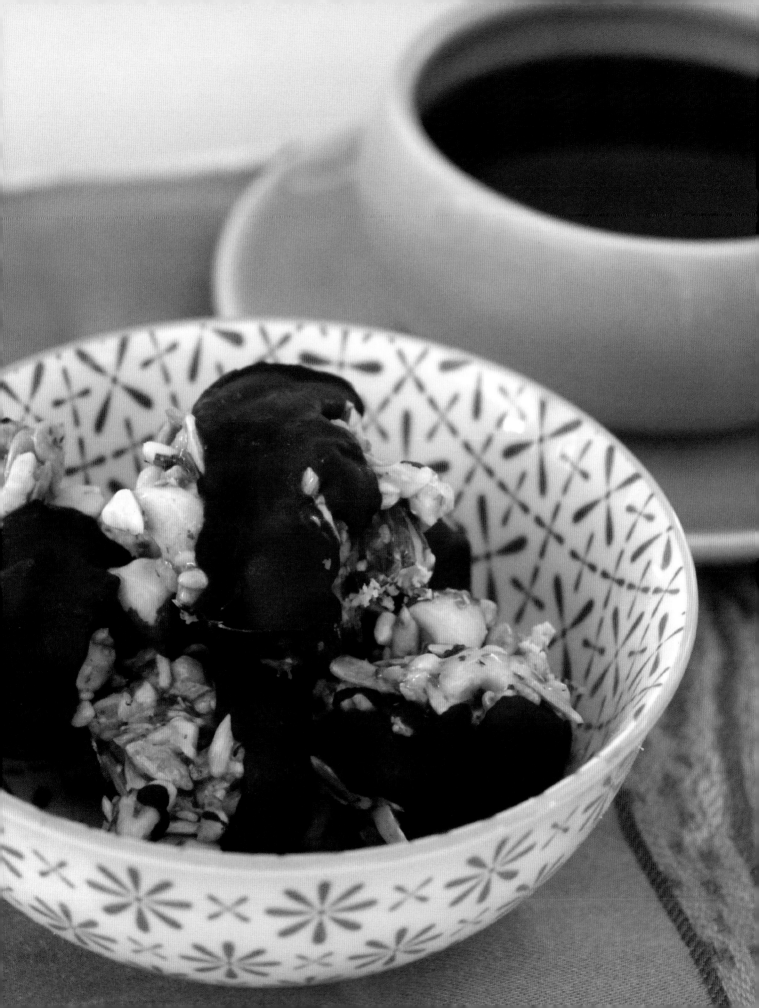

Sunflower Butter & Jelly Cookies (vegan and peanut-free)
Makes 20 cookies

These cookies are a great baking project for kids with peanut allergies. Get creative with fun designs and different jelly flavors to give the cookies personal flair!

ingredients
2 flaxseed eggs (2 Tablespoons flaxseed meal plus 6 Tablespoons warm water)
1 cup Gluten-Free All-Purpose Baking Mix (see page 144)
½ teaspoon baking powder
¼ teaspoon baking soda
½ teaspoon sea salt
1 cup creamy sunflower butter
¼ cup vegan butter, at room temperature
¾ cup granulated sugar
¼ cup light brown sugar, firmly packed
3 Tablespoons and 1 teaspoon jelly
¼ cup and 2 Tablespoons powdered sugar
1½ Tablespoons dairy-free milk (almond, coconut, hemp etc.)

directions
Preheat the oven to 350°F. Prepare 2 baking sheets by lining with parchment paper or baking mats, then set aside.

Mix together the flaxseed meal and water in a small bowl and allow it to sit for a few minutes.

In a small bowl, stir together the flour, baking powder, baking soda, and salt. Set aside.

In a large bowl, mix ¾ cup of the sunflower butter with the vegan butter on medium speed. Add the granulated sugar and brown sugar and beat until smooth, about 5 minutes. Beat in the flaxseed mixture until incorporated. Stir in the reserved flour mixture until just combined.

Drop the dough 2 inches apart on two prepared baking sheets. Using the back of a melon baller or your thumb, gently dent the center of each cookie. Spoon about ½ teaspoon of jelly into each center. Bake until lightly golden, about 12 minutes. Allow cookies to sit on sheet for 5 minutes before transferring to a rack to cool completely.

In a small bowl, beat together the remaining ¼ cup of sunflower butter and the powdered sugar. Whisk in milk, a little at a time, until the frosting reaches a good consistency for piping. Using a resealable sandwich bag with a tiny corner snipped off, pipe the frosting over the cookies.

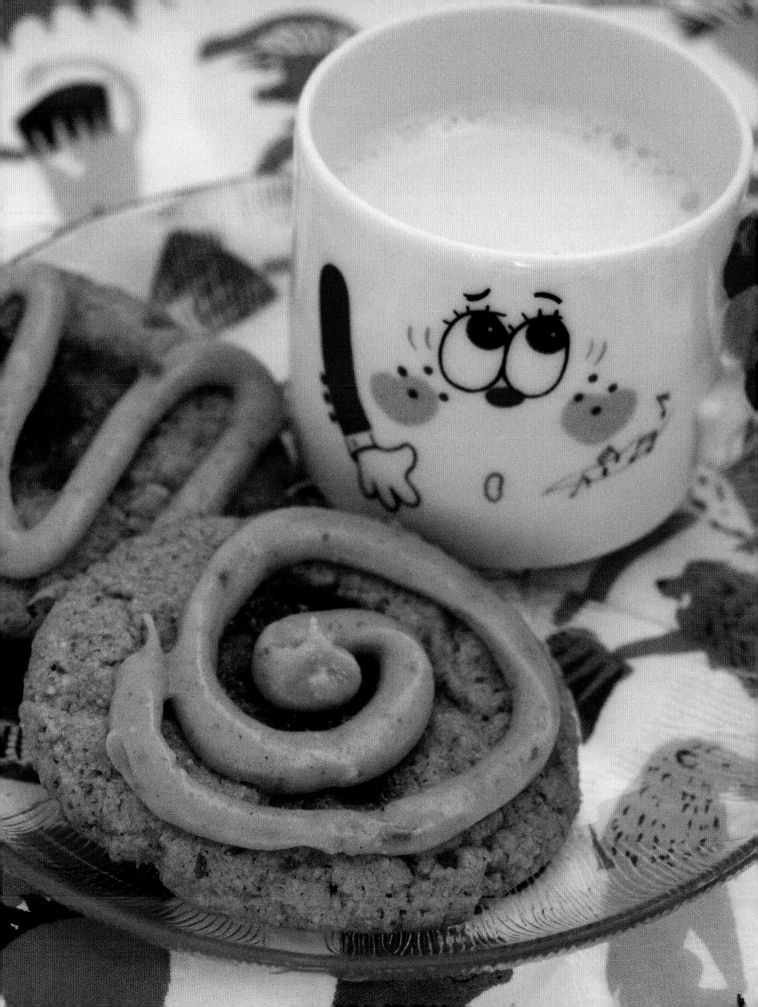

Peanut Butter & Banana Cupcakes (vegan)

Makes 30 mini cupcakes

Who doesn't love an old-fashioned peanut butter and banana sandwich? These cupcakes bring a childhood favorite to life, using butter, milk, and egg substitutes to keep 'em vegan.

ingredients

cake

2 flaxseed eggs (2 Tablespoons flaxseed meal plus 6 Tablespoons warm water)
1 cup granulated vegan sugar
2 small (about 1 cup) overripe bananas, mashed
½ cup safflower or grapeseed oil
1 cup Gluten-Free All-Purpose Baking Mix (see page 144)
1 teaspoon baking powder
½ teaspoon baking soda
1 teaspoon ground cinnamon
¼ teaspoon sea salt

frosting

1½ cups powdered sugar
¼ cup dairy-free milk
¼ cup creamy peanut butter
¼ cup vegetable or palm shortening
½ teaspoon pure vanilla extract

directions

For cake:

Preheat oven to 350° F. Prepare mini muffin pans by lining with muffin cups or brushing with safflower oil. Mix together the flaxseed meal and water in a small bowl and allow it to sit for a few minutes.

Using a standing mixer or medium bowl with hand mixer, combine vegan sugar, bananas, and oil. Add flaxseed mixture. Combine flour, baking powder, baking soda, cinnamon, and sea salt in a separate medium bowl. Slowly add flour combination to the wet ingredients, mixing until combined. Fill each muffin cup ¾ full. Bake for 25–26 minutes until golden brown, or until a toothpick inserted into the center comes out clean.

For frosting:

In a medium bowl, beat together powdered sugar, milk, peanut butter, vegetable shortening, and vanilla until smooth. Smooth or pipe frosting on top of each cooled cupcake.

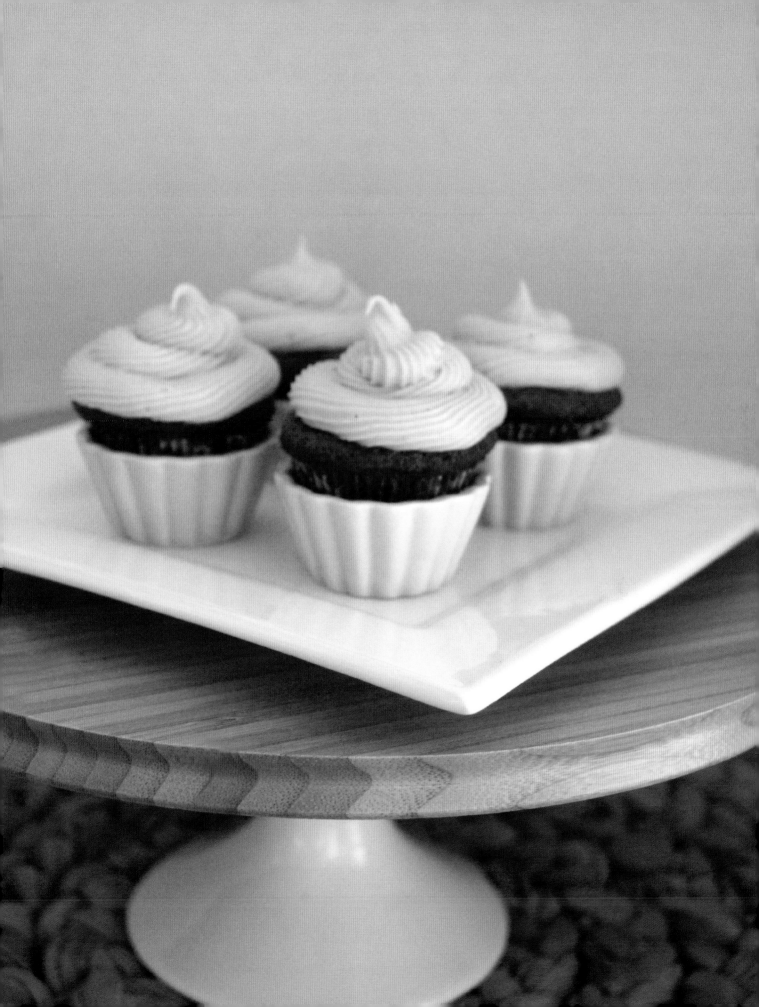

Chapter Three:
The Lifestyle

let's get physical

Take-'Em-Anywhere Yoga Poses

4 Poses for Reducing Head Pain

Drool-Worthy Sleepy Time Yoga
   Sequence

On Running

15-Minute Cardio Pilates

5 Ballet-Inspired Exercises for a Perky Booty

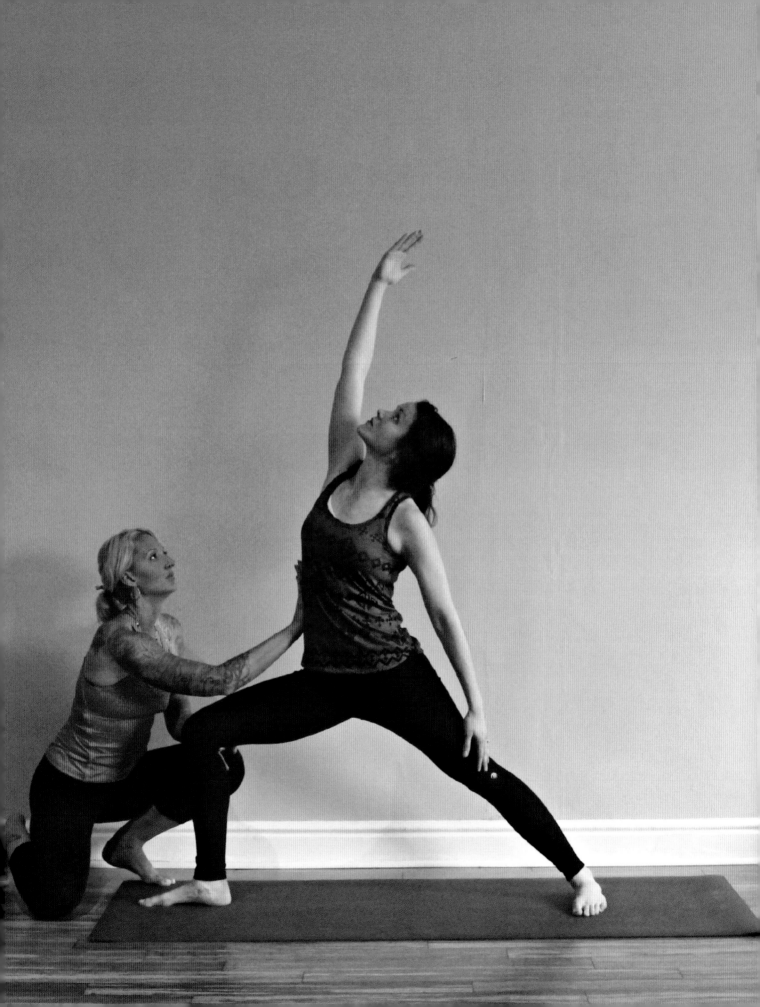

Take-'Em-Anywhere Yoga Poses

LA Finfinger is one of those people whose very presence can make you feel as if you are basking in glittery sunshine. As a yoga instructor, writer, and friend, she always seems to be working with the purpose of creating peace and happiness for those who surround her. That's why I knew she was just the sweet pea who could design simple yoga poses for people to do anywhere. Whether you need a quick break from the office or a simple stretch in your hotel room, these poses will give you the bit of Zen you are seeking—no equipment required.

Paripurna Navasana – Boat Pose

Sit on the floor with your legs out long in front of you. Keep your chest lifted as your lift your legs. Feel the low belly engage. Arms can reach forward with the palms faceup or palms facing the thighs. Keep the top of the head lifting. Allow your body to make a wide V. (If this is too much, then bend both knees and allow the shins to be parallel with the floor.) Continue to let the top of the head lift so that the spine lengthens and the core stays engaged.

LA says: "You will feel the heat building. Allow it to burn off some of the stress or fatigue of the day. Start by counting to five or ten. After that, continue to build until you are holding the pose for a minute."

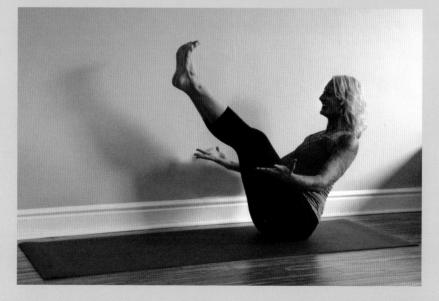

Uttanasana – Rag Doll Pose

Stand with your feet about hips' width apart from each other. Fold forward at the waist. Place each hand into the crook of the opposite elbow. Let the top of your head move toward the floor.

LA says: "This is a sweet pose to reward yourself after sitting all day. Allow yourself to let go of tension by gently turning the head from side to side to release the neck. Let your back relax into this by bending your knees as much as you need. Imagine your whole workday sliding off the top of your head."

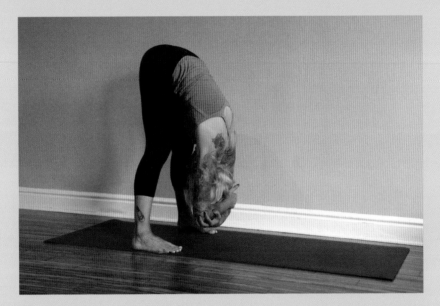

Crescent Lunge

This dynamic and warming pose gets the blood circulating. It allows for all parts of the body to activate!

Begin on your hands and knees, keeping your wrists underneath your shoulders and your knees in line with your hips. Inhale as you tuck your toes and exhale to lift your hips, coming into an upside down "V" shape (downward facing dog). Transition into Crescent Lunge by stepping your right foot between your hands. Stay on the ball of the back left foot as you reach your arms toward the sky. Keep your right knee bent. Tuck your tailbone toward your pubic bone to lengthen through the lower back. As the arms reach, allow the shoulders to relax away from the ears. Take 5–10 deep breaths here. After the last breath, place the hands to either side of the right foot and step the right foot back to meet the left in downward facing dog. Repeat on the left!

LA says: "This pose allows the center of the chest to lift and open. Imagine that you're opening up to some moments of new possibility as you breathe in and out through your nose with calm, steady breath."

When you are ready to come back to standing, use your inhale to lift halfway. Use your exhale to lift back to standing.

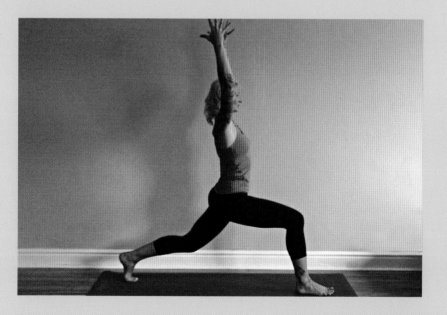

Prasarita Padottanasana – Wide-Legged Forward Bend

From standing, take your feet out wide. Allow the feet to be parallel.

LA says: "Some people, myself included, find it slightly more comfortable to turn the heels out a bit wider than the toes."

Catch a hold of the hips and with an inhale look toward the ceiling. Exhale as you fold forward. Allow your hands to drop to the floor (or yoga mat). Let the top of your head reach toward the floor.

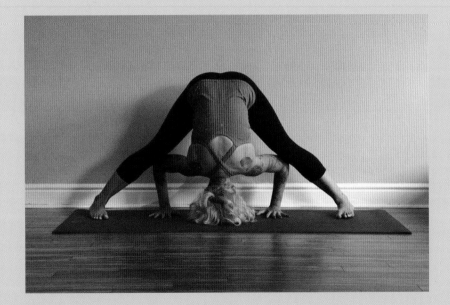

LA Finfinger is a Pittsburgh-based yoga instructor. You can discover more of her dazzling beauty at lafinfinger.com.

Chatting with LA

Q: If there was one thing you could tell your teenage self, what would it be?

A: It all works out and it all falls apart. You will be okay.

You will feel pain that you have never felt in your worst nightmare. You will also know joy that is beyond description.

At 34, you will have grown into the nose that you swore you would fix as soon as you could afford it.

You will never look like all of the other girls. (This will be to your benefit.)

You will never learn to hold your tongue. (This will sometimes be to your detriment.)

The lyrics that you heard from Baz Luhrmann in your teenage years will ring just as true in your thirties: "The race is long and in the end, it's only with yourself." Oh and you were right about the calculus—you won't need it in the long run (so far). But study up on the public speaking—it'll come in more handy than you yet know.

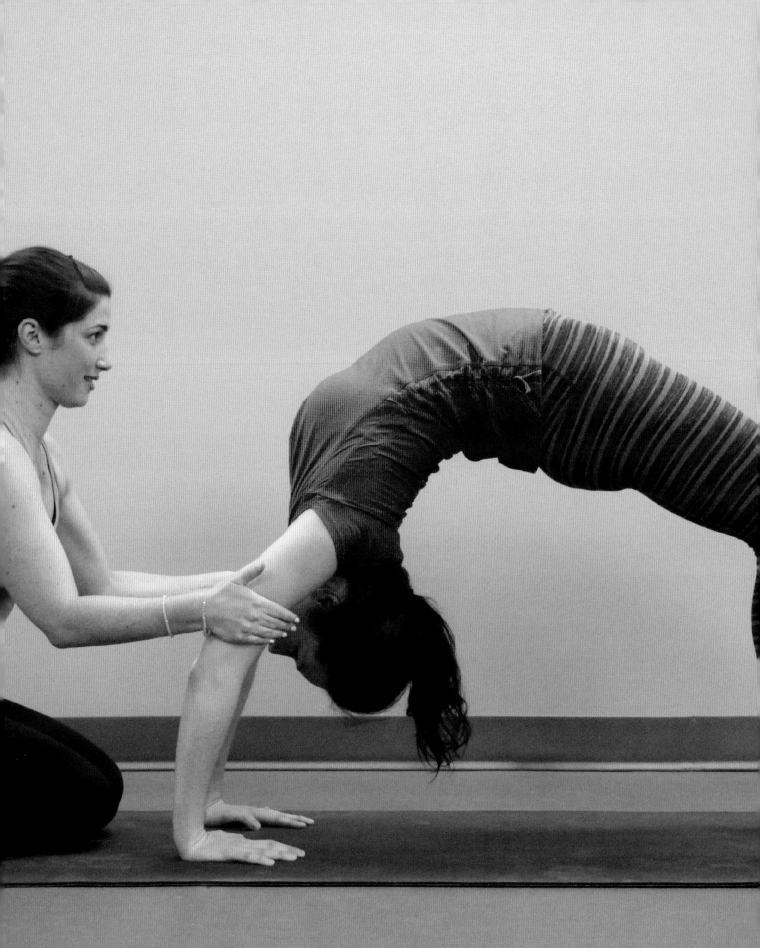

4 Yoga Poses for Reducing Head Pain

I'm fairly confident that the sound of **Anna Gilbert Zupon's** voice could make me feel calm on even the most stressful days. Unlike the stuffy associations some people tie to yoga, Anna's practice is one that somehow manages to make a student feel centered, all while keeping a smile splayed across the face throughout the duration of bending and chanting. In fact, it's not unlike Anna to put a halt to an unfocused class and hit the mat to talk about some better ways to approach a practice.

Here, Anna shares with you some poses that can help ease a tense neck and shoulders and even provide relief to common migraine headaches. Do the whole sequence for the best results, or pick your favorite pose and get relaxed.

Props needed: blanket

Constructive Rest Pose:

Rest on your back and support your head with a small pillow or rolled blanket so that it is slightly elevated. Separate your feet so that they are as wide as your hips and let your knees gently fall in toward one another to touch. Take a moment to adjust the distance between your feet so that your knees can rest on one another without any effort in the legs. You can place your hands on your abdomen or let the arms rest by your sides, whatever feels most comfortable. Allow your spine to maintain its natural curvature. You don't need to do anything muscularly; in fact you are giving the body an opportunity to undo. Breathe here for 5–10 minutes.

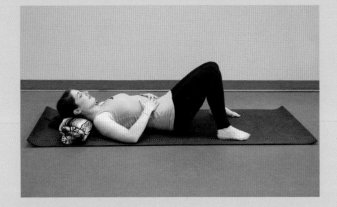

Janu Sirsasana – Head-to-Knee Pose

From a seated position reach both legs out straight, then bend your right leg and open the knee out to the side, bringing the sole of the right foot to meet the inner left thigh. Bring your fingertips to the ground to frame your left leg. Inhale to lengthen all four sides of your waist and exhale to twist to the left in the direction of your straight leg. Continue to use each inhale to find length and space and each exhale to revolve your torso and fold forward.

Stay for 1–2 minutes and then repeat on the second side with the position of the legs reversed, revolving in the opposite direction.

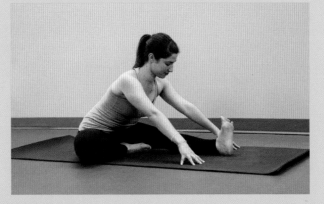

Setu Bandha Sarvangasana – Bridge Pose

Lie down on your back and bend your knees so that your feet come to the floor near your hips and your arms come to your sides. Begin to spin your arms by rolling the outer arms down and letting the chest lift. Press into the upper outer arms and down through the feet to lift your hips. Keep lifting as the shoulder blades draw together and the chest opens. You can interlace your hands underneath your back for leverage or keep the arms by your sides. Relax the neck and jaw and stay for 30 seconds to 1 minute. Use an exhale to lower down to your back. Repeat a second time switching the interlace of your hands.

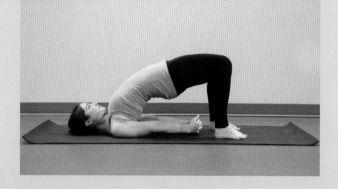

Reclined Spinal Twist

From your back with your knees bent and feet flat on the mat, pick your hips up and shift them a few inches to the right. Draw both knees into your chest and let them drop over to the left side. Reach your arms wide into a T position. Your gaze can go over your right shoulder or stay up toward the ceiling. Inhale and imagine the breath spreading wide into your wing span, fingertip to fingertip, and exhale to allow the breath to return back to your sternum at the center of your chest. Take 5–10 breaths before coming up to center. Hug your knees into your chest and place the feet down on the mat to shift your hips left and twist to the right for 5–10 breaths.

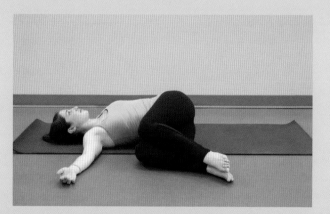

Anna Gilbert Zupon, RYT, is a Pittsburgh-based instructor and YogaWorks teacher trainer who enjoys providing her students with a playful yet focused environment where they discover personal empowerment. Learn more at www.AnnaGilbertZupon.com

Drool-Worthy Sleepy Time Yoga Sequence

Ask me any time, day or night, and I will tell you **Maggie Ryan** is one of the few people on this planet whose mere presence can make anyone grin. She is one of those people who emanate all things wonderful—a warm smile, listening ear, or simply a goofy story. It is going to sound cliché, but I will say it anyway: She absolutely glows.

Here, Maggie helps us get down to business with easing our bodies into rest mode. I don't know about you, but I have a hard time shutting down at the end of the day. I swear I hit the pillow and that's the moment my brain decides to shift into full gear, making lists and lists of things to do the next day.

"Our bodies are so overstressed and overstimulated, meaning we are constantly in a state of 'fight or flight,'" Maggie said. "When the sympathetic nervous system is activated, blood in the body rushes to the extremities to prepare for either battle or escape."

Maggie explained that this perpetual sympathetic response makes it very difficult for the body to fully digest, rest, and heal. The parasympathetic nervous system (or relaxation mode) can only be gently coaxed into activation. When the parasympathetic nervous system is activated, the heart rate decreases, the body relaxes, and intestinal activity increases.

"A good way to cajole the relaxation response is to practice restorative poses," Maggie said. "Fewer poses with longer holds can feel simply scrumptious— even drool-worthy."

Ready to catch some shut-eye? Me too.

Props needed: bolster/pillows, blankets, and yoga strap/belt

Restorative Upavishta Konasana – Wide-Angle Seated Forward Fold

Extend your legs into a gentle straddle position. There is absolutely no need to pancake your body all the way down to the floor. Instead, bring the floor up to you by either resting on a combined stack of bolsters, pillows, and/or blankets. Drape your torso over the stack, and let your forehead rest atop the pile or turn your cheek to the side. If you have tight hamstrings, or you notice it is hard to sit up straight initially in the straddle, place either one or two blankets under your buttocks.

Hold for 3 to 5 minutes. If you turned your cheek to one side, make sure you turn your head the opposite way halfway through the pose.

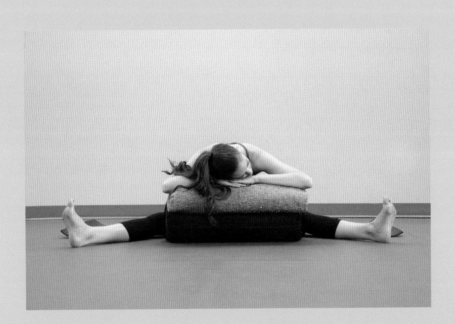

Viparita Karani – Legs-Up-the-Wall Pose
Create approximately a hip-sized loop in a strap or belt, and move the buckle so that it is not touching your skin. Let your legs fall out into the strap. You may feel a delightful release in your lower back. When your feet start to fall asleep, you can bend your knees and place your feet flat on the wall. If you have tight hamstrings you can always bend your knees and rest your calves on your couch or a chair.

Hold for 3–5 minutes. (Various contraindications to this pose include: eye health issues, pregnancy, heart conditions, hiatal hernia, and very high or low blood pressure.)

Maggie says: "This gentle inversion is a gem. You can simply extend your legs up the wall, and practice the pose sans props. My favorite Viparita variation involves placing a strap or belt around the ankles and letting the legs fall out into the strap."

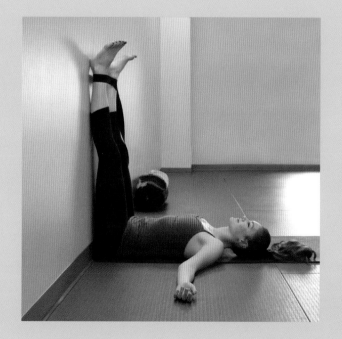

Supta Baddha Konasana – Reclined Bound Angle Pose

Bring the soles of your feet together to touch, and let your knees fall out to the side. Trifold a blanket (so that it is long and skinny) and place it over top of your feet and underneath of your ankles. Rest on your back, and bring your hands either out to the sides (palms facing up) or on top of your stomach. If you have tender knees or inner thighs, you can always place blankets or pillows underneath your knees.

Hold for 3 to 5 minutes.

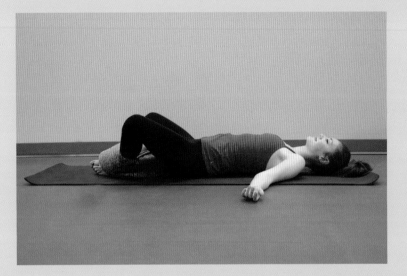

Savasana

Lie on your back and extend your legs straight. You can place a bolster or blankets underneath your knees to provide an extra release for the lower back. Give yourself plenty of time in savasana.

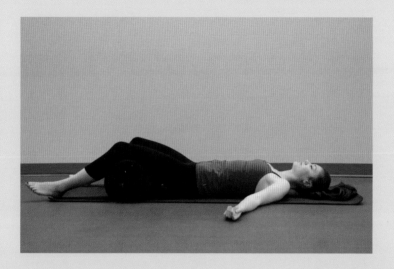

Maggie Ryan completed her first Vinyasa teacher training in 2010. In 2012, she went on to complete her 200-hour training with Chrissy Carter at YogaWorks NYC. Maggie teaches an alignment-based class with fluid yet intuitive sequences. She uses humor to create a lighter practice, and as a reminder to stay grounded in the present moment. When she's not teaching, Maggie Ryan works as an actor both onstage and on-screen. Find out more about Maggie Ryan at www.maggiefinnryan.com

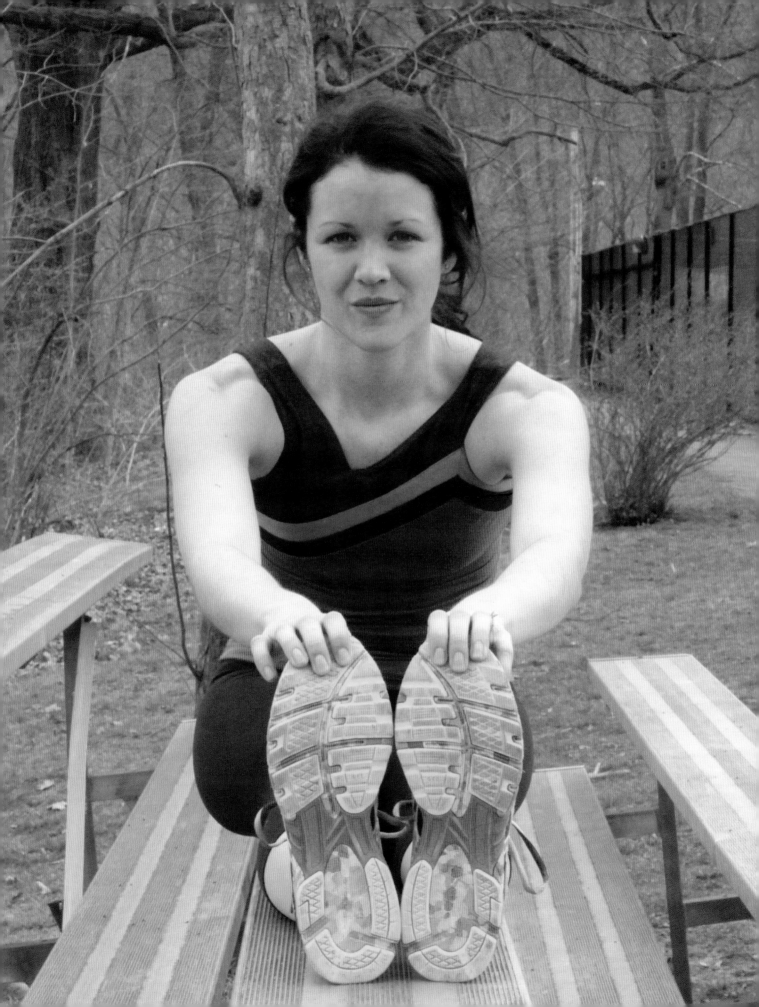

on running

I started running when I was just 12 years old. Coming from two parents who ran cross-country in their high school and college days, it was only a matter of time before I joined them in their favorite outdoor activity. One morning during the summer before my venture into 7th grade, I watched as my mom laced up her running shoes.

"Can I come with you?" I asked. She cheerfully nodded and the rest is history.

But that's not to say the last 17 or so years have been filled with running bliss. No, as a matter of fact, the average runner will tell you that so many of those days are filled with a range of body aches and emotions that *literally* feel like an uphill battle.

But there's just something about that oft-touted runner's high that keeps us coming back for more. Time and time again I have found myself mid-run and swearing to a higher power that if I just make it through that run, I will never again hit the pavement.

Still, I do. Because there's nothing like taking that last stride. Nothing like crossing the finish line. And no other sweat that can compare to that of a solid run.

Here are a few of my favorite running tips, learned throughout the years and stolen, of course, from my favorite coach—my mom.

1. **Have a side cramp?** Try inhaling, then exhaling with force through parted lips. Feel the air pressing against your lips as it makes its way out of your mouth. Continue this until your cramps begin to alleviate.
2. **Use your arms.** I can't tell you how many times I've seen runners trucking down a path with their arms hanging limply by their sides. Use 'em people!

If you haven't been doing so, then it will be hard to get used to at first. However, pumping your arms can help take you up the toughest of hills—even when your legs just don't wanna.

3. **Relax your face.** It sounds silly, but we carry so much tension in our faces. Next time you're out for a run, notice if your eyebrows are furrowed or you are overly squinting your eyes. Try relaxing those muscles and notice that you instantly feel more at ease.

4. **Use your booty!** Out to conquer some tough hills? Put your brain in your booty and feel the work coming from the muscles just under your bum cheeks. How do you think runners get those muscular behinds?

5. **Shrink your stride.** Running gurus, like Jeff Galloway, say the most efficient stride is one that mimics a shuffle with your feet hovering just above the ground. As long as your foot is lifted enough to avoid tripping over uneven pavement or a rock, then you are doing the necessary work. A stride that is too long or high can lead to injury.

Implementing the Run-to-the-Next-Mailbox Method

When I first began running, my momma taught me to "just work toward the next mailbox." What she meant was that when I was running, it was much easier to say, "OK, I just have to make it to that mailbox down the street, and then I can stop" as opposed to thinking about the run in its entirety. What I found was that I would often keep running to just one more "mailbox," completing a few miles before I realized it.

These small running goals make the task of lacing up our shoes seem more attainable. If you've never gone for a run or brisk walk, then the idea of keeping it up for miles seems daunting enough that it could deter you from venturing out at all.

But what if I told you all you had to do was run for three minutes? Two minutes? One minute?

It might make the task seem a little more doable, right? Here I test two different plans to prove that running in intervals can be just as effective—and heart pumping—as running for consistent miles. In both 45-minute workouts, I plugged in my current weight (approximately 127 pounds) and age (29 years old). Take a look at the results.

Option #1:

Minutes	Speed	Incline
0:00 - 4:00	4.4	2.5%
4:00-7:00	6.5	2.5%
7:00-9:00	4.4	2.5%
9:00-12:00	6.6	2.5%
12:00-14:00	4.4	2.5%
14:00-17:00	6.6	2.5%
17:00-19:00	4.4	2.5%
19:00-22:00	6.8	2.5%
22:00-24:00	4.4	2.5%
24:00-27:00	6.8	2.5%
27:00-29:00	4.4	2.5%
29:00-32:00	7.0	2.5%
32:00-34:00	4.4	2.5%
34:00-37:00	7.2	2.5%
37:00-39:00	4.4	2.5%
39:00-41:00	7.4	2.5%
41:00-42:00	7.6	2.5%
42:00-43:00	4.2	2.5%
43:00-44:00	4.0	2.5%
44:00-45:00	3.8	2.5%

Option #2:

Minutes	Speed	Incline
0:00-4:00	4.4	1%
4:00-42:00	7.0	1%
42:00-43:00	4.2	1%
43:00-44:00	4.0	1%
44:00-45:00	3.8	1%

RESULTS

Option #1: I traveled 4.3 miles and burned 443 calories.

Option #2: I traveled 4.9 miles and burned 500 calories.

You know what that means? These results show that if I had run for a consistent 38 minutes as opposed to doing run-walk intervals, then I would have traveled approximately 6/10 of a mile farther and burned approximately 50 more calories.

Guess what I say to that? Eat one less cookie, laugh at your favorite comedian or, hell, have sex to knock off that additional 50 calories. If it means conquering a workout as opposed to feeling defeated, then it is undoubtedly a win-win situation.

need to scale it back?

Take the incline down to 1 percent (always keep treadmill at a slight incline to mimic natural ground surfaces and avoid injury) or decrease the running speed across the board. For instance, if you take the first running interval from 6.5 to 6.0, then each running interval should be decreased by .5 miles per hour. As you build strength, you can begin to increase the speed.

ready to take it up a notch?

Intersperse hills throughout the workout, increasing the inline a bit during the last minute or two of a running interval. For example, if you are running at 7.0 miles per hour for three minutes, then the last minute of the interval might be done on an increased incline, such as 5 percent as opposed to the original 2.5 percent. These small changes will increase calorie burn and keep a workout from feeling ho-hum.

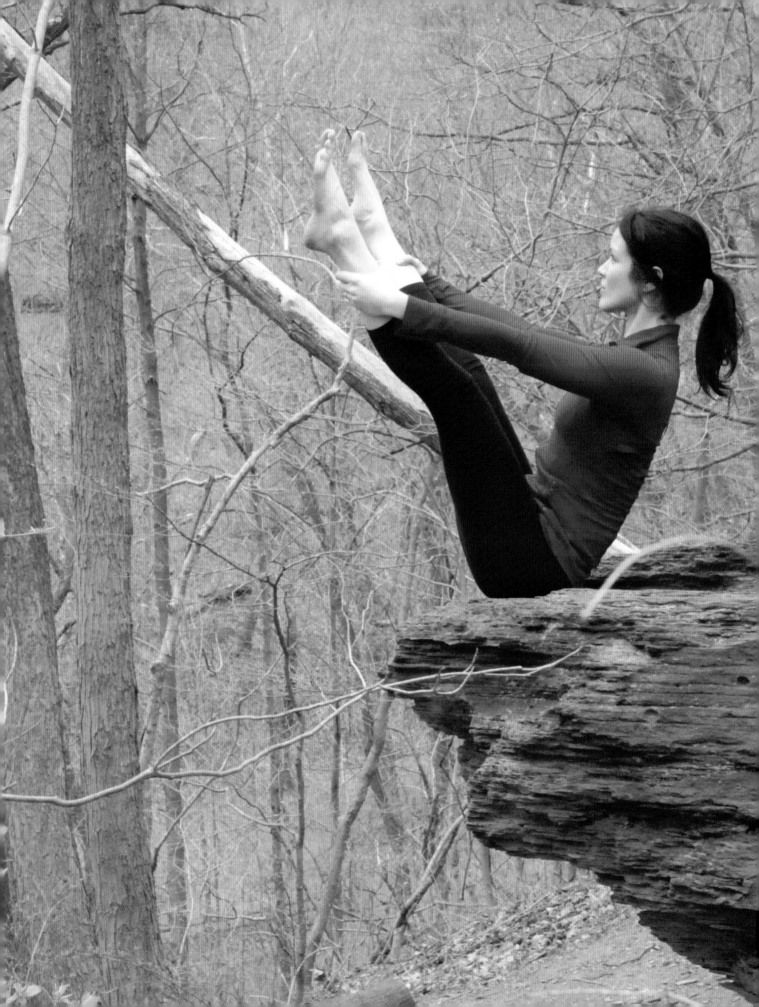

15-Minute Cardio Pilates Workout

Do this cardio Pilates workout while watching television or waiting for dinner to cook in the oven. Perform the whole circuit once. Have more time? Do it twice for a longer sweat session!

Warm-up: 1 minute of jumping jacks

Crisscross

Lie on your back with your hands behind your head and your knees bent into your chest (a). Extend your left leg out long in front of you and twist your upper body until left elbow touches right knee (b). Switch sides, inhaling and exhaling with each twist. Imagine that your center is anchored to the mat, so you don't rock from hip to hip. Complete 8–10 sets (16–20 repetitions each side).

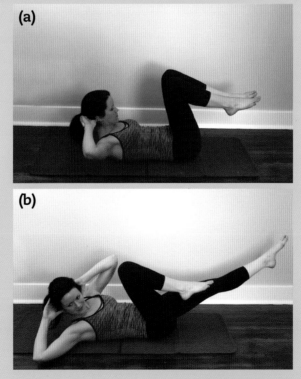

Single Leg Stretch

Sit on the center of your mat with your knees bent. Place your left hand on the outside of your left ankle and right hand on your knee; roll your back onto the mat, bringing your bent leg with you and extending your opposite leg straight in front of you (a). Inhale and allow navel to sink into spine. Exhale and switch legs, bringing right hand to right ankle and left hand to knee (b); that is one set. Complete 8–10 sets.

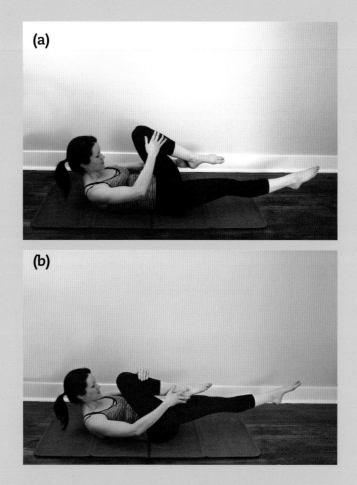

Cardio burst: 1 minute of high knees or running in place

Bridge with Leg Kick

Lie on your back with feet hips' width apart and planted firmly on the mat; arms are long at sides. Squeeze your buttocks up off the mat and raise your hips (a). Pull your navel deep into your spine and stretch one leg out long in front of you (b). Kick it up to the ceiling (c), exhaling as you bring it back, lowering your leg to position (b), then repeat 5–8 times. Lower the leg to its original position (a), then repeat on other side. When complete, lower back down to mat, one vertebrae at a time. Pull knees into chest for a lower back stretch.

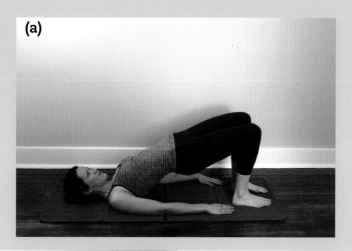

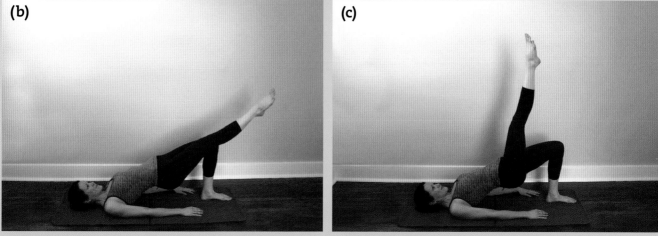

Rolling Like a Ball

Sit toward the front of your mat with knees bent into your chest, heels together, knees open, and hands on ankles (a). Scoop belly by sinking navel deep into spine, maintaining eye contact with navel (b). Inhale as you roll back (c) and exhale as you roll forward. Each time you roll up it is important to balance on your tailbone; do not allow feet to touch mat. Repeat 6–8 times.

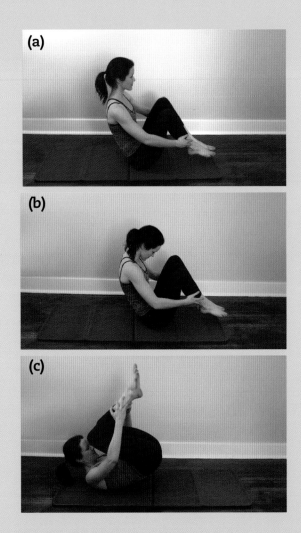

Cardio burst: 1 minute of mountain climbers

Push-ups

Stand at the back of your mat with feet and legs hips' width apart. Inhale, pulling your navel into your spine, then exhale rolling head down toward mat until palms are touching—or close to touching!—the mat. Walk hands forward into a plank position (a). Modify by bringing knees to the mat. Perform 3–5 push-ups by bending and straightening elbows with elbows close to sides (b). Complete 2–3 sets, resting in child's pose between each set.

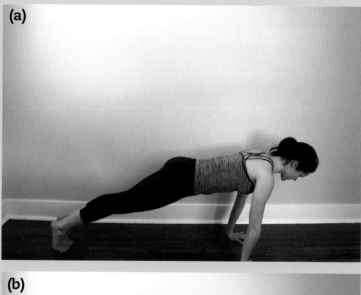

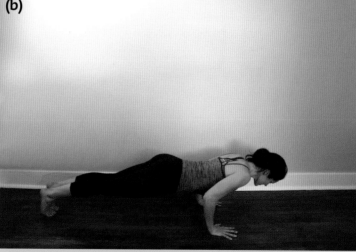

Mermaid Stretch

Sit on mat with left hand at your side on the mat and right arm up toward the ceiling, palm facing upward. Right leg should be bent in with foot pressing against the left thigh and left thigh is bent behind (a). Be sure hips are squared and facing forward, and you can feel the bottom part of your glutes (proper term: Sitz bones) on the mat. Reach right arm up and over the body, bending your right side while keeping left hand on the mat for support (b). Feel the stretch from the tips of your right fingers all the way through the hip. Hips should remain unmoving in order to fully reap the benefits of this stretch. Return to starting position and reverse arms, reaching left arm over to the right side. Return to starting position to complete one repetition. Repeat for a total of 6 to 8 repetitions. Switch sides and repeat.

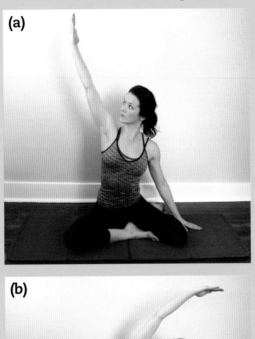

Tip! Set small, achievable goals. Knock out your workout one minute at a time. At the end of each minute, ask yourself, "*Do I have another minute in me?*" If so, then rock it out, sweet pea.

5 Ballet-Inspired Exercises for a Perky Booty

Misty Lynne Cauthen, owner of Dragonfly Pilates, is one of the first people I met during my Pilates training. At the time, I was 16 years old and I had no idea what to expect from this training. Then, Misty walked into the studio, and I knew she was about to show me. Throughout that time, I learned how her military-trained father taught her to do push-ups (inhale on your way down, use the exhale to bring you back up) and that, despite her tough exterior, she had a heart meant for making people feel good about their bodies.

Here Misty shares with you some of her tried-and-true moves for getting your behind in tip-top shape. All you need is a chair!

Diamond Pelvic Press

Start Position: Lie on back, with knees bent, feet flat on floor (with heels at least one foot length from rear-end) and heels pressed together in a 10 and 2 o'clock position. Scoop belly in, use abdominals to lift hips to waistband (a).

Movement Sequence: Exhale, engaging glutes, pressing hips toward ceiling (about 1–3 inches). Repeat 2 sets, 6–8 repetitions each (b).

Feel the Movement: Imagine you have a sleeping baby in the scoop of your belly. As you press your pelvis up, try not to roll the baby off!

Where's the Work? Gluteals, abdominals, inner and outer thighs

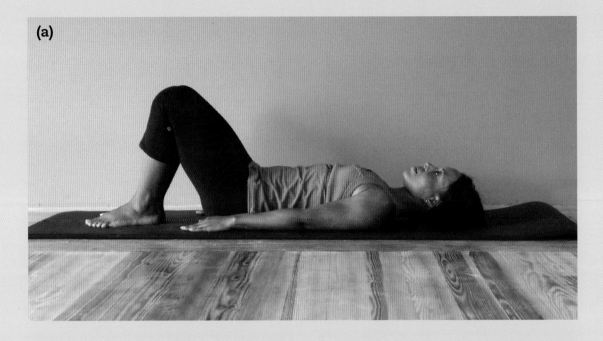

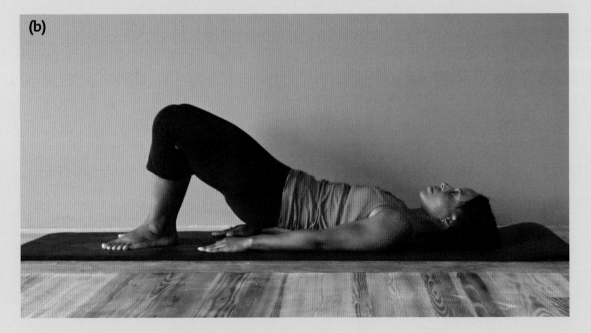

THE GLUTEN-FREE REVOLUTION

Diagonal Booty Drop

Start Position: Lie on back, with knees bent, feet flat on floor (with heels at least one foot length from rear-end) and parallel. Feet and knees should be in-line with center of hips. Pelvis is pressed up to a bridge position.

Movement Sequence: Keeping spine straight, inhale and engage glutes while lowering pelvis to the right side of the mat. Exhale to return to start position. Repeat, lowering pelvis to left side of mat. Repeat 2 sets, 6–8 repetitions each.

Where's the Work? Gluteals, abdominals, lateral hips, hamstrings

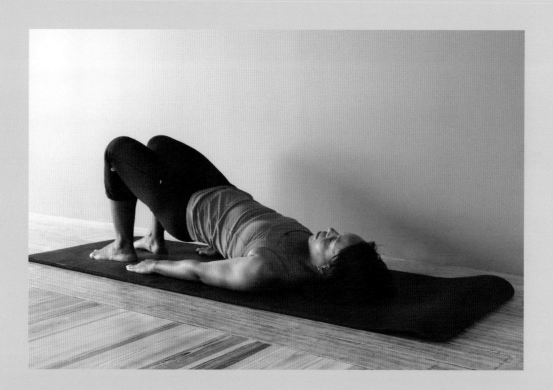

Side Leg Raise

Start Position: Stand with one hand on chair or countertop, with feet parallel (a).

Movement Sequence: Inhale to lift outside leg to a 45° angle, standing straight on the standing leg (b). Exhale to return to start position. Continue for a total of 6–8 repetitions, then repeat on other leg. Complete two sets total.

Feel the Movement: Imagine pushing a boulder away from your leg with the outside of your ankle. Pull your leg back to start with resistance and control.

Where's the Work? Gluteals, lateral hips, inner thighs

Bonus: Repeat same move, this time with feet in a "V" position (heels together, toes turned out to 10 and 2 o'clock position). Complete 2 sets of 6–8 repetitions on each leg.

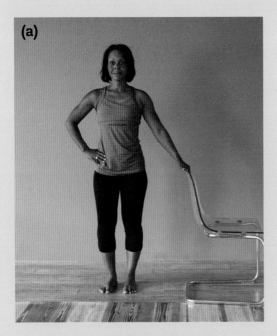
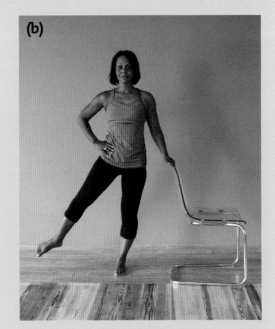

Side Leg Scissor

Start Position: Stand with one hand on chair or countertop, with feet in a "V" (heels together, toes turned out to 10 and 2 o'clock position).

Movement Sequence: Inhale to flex right foot and lift leg to a 45° angle (a). Exhale to bring the leg down to the front, with the heel touching the left toes (b). Inhale to lift leg back to starting position, then exhale to bring right leg behind standing leg, right toe tapping left heel. Return to starting position and continue sequence for a total of 6–8 repetitions. Switch sides and repeat on left leg. Complete two sets on each leg.

Feel the Movement: Imagine you're using your legs to squeeze the water out of a towel with your inner thighs. As the leg comes forward, feel like the inner and outer thighs are moving it—not the foot! And try not to lean forward or back—good posture is a virtue (and a booty-buster!).

Where's the Work? Inner and outer thighs, lateral hip, glutes (on standing leg)

Bonus: Repeat same move, this time with feet in a parallel position. Complete 1 set of 6–8 repetitions on each leg.

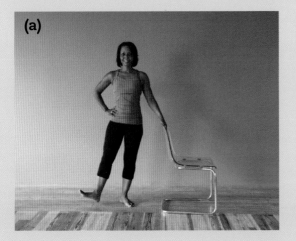
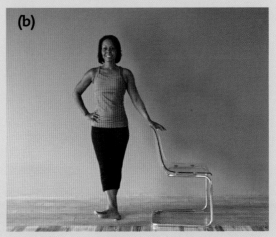

Slo-Mo Donkey Kick

Start Position: Stand with two hands on chair or countertop, with feet in a v (heels together, toes turned out to 10 and 2 o'clock position).

Movement Sequence: Lift right leg straight back about 2–4 inches, without leaning forward. Keep the foot rotated to the 2 o'clock position (a). Bend the knee, flexing the foot and curling the heel toward the right glute (b). Extend the knee, pushing from the cheek through the heel. Complete 6–8 repetitions, then repeat on left leg. Complete 2 sets on each leg.

Feel the Movement: Imagine you have a spring attached to your working heel and your opposite glute. As you curl the heel, think of resisting the coiling of the spring. As you extend, keep the thigh still and really work through the entire leg to stretch the spring.

Where's the Work? Outer thighs, glutes, hamstrings, abdominals

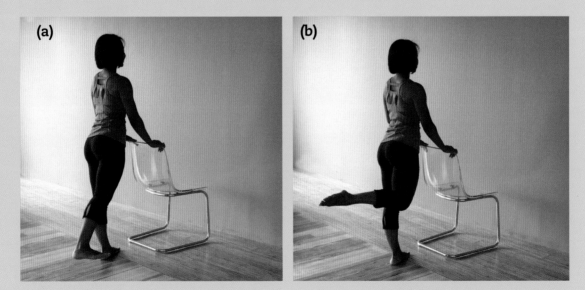

Misty Lynne Cauthen, Certified Master Trainer and Owner of Dragonfly Pilates, has been a certified Pilates instructor since 2001. Since discovering the benefits of Pilates, Misty has made it her mission to bring the healing, invigorating, and uplifting effects of the program to her clients and friends. Learn more at dragonflypilates.com.

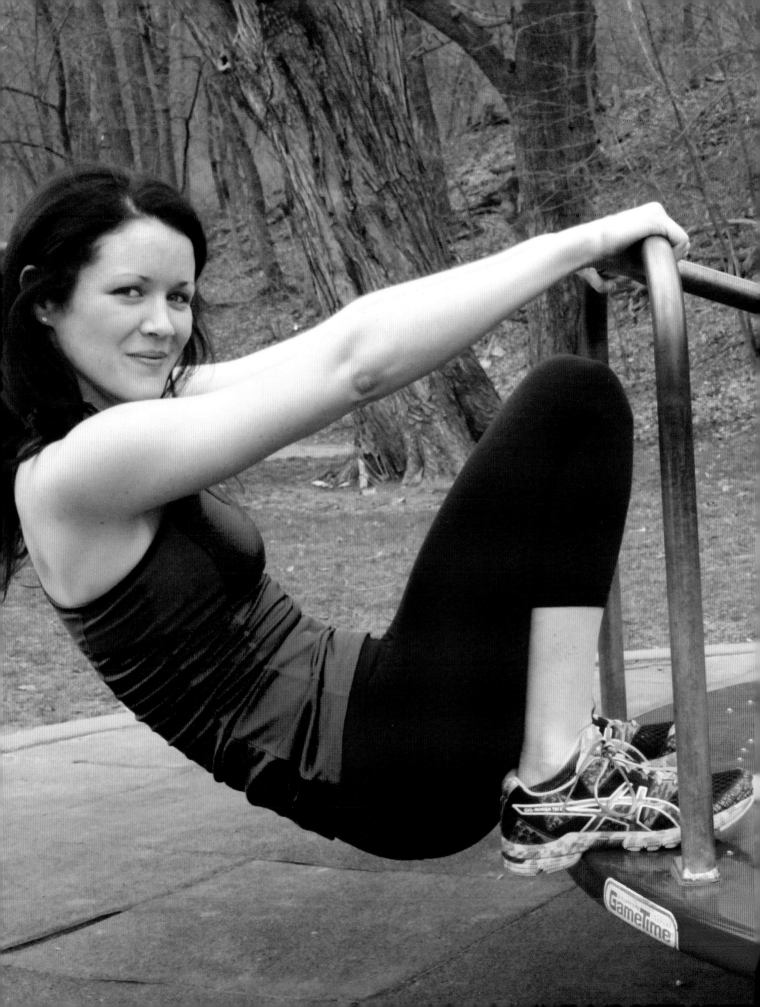

mirror, mirror

I'm a true believer that gorgeous, glowing skin is made in the kitchen and a toned body is made with some serious sweat action. But that's not to say that a girl can't love putting on some beauty products every now and then. Get the details on gluten-free beauty goodies, plus DIY tips for making at-home treatments.

Gluten-Free Beauty

Sure, we're always looking for gluten in our food and drinks. But what about when the sneaky little guy makes its way into our beauty goodies? Some people say it's a wash, others say you have to watch your gorgeous back when it comes to choosing primping products. I say, "Why take the risk?" Here are a few of my picks, varying from everyday budget options to those you might want to scoop up before a hot date.

face cleanser

Desert Essence Gentle Nourishing Organic Cleanser *desertessence.com*

Gluten Free Beauty's Exfoliating Olive Oil Cleanser *glutenfreebeauty.com*

lotion

Desert Essence Coconut Hand & Body Lotion *desertessence.com*

Kiss My Face Vitamin A&E Lotion *kissmyface.com*

lip balm, gloss & lipstick

Mineral Fusion Lip Gloss *mineralfusion.com*

EOS Lip Balm *evolutionofsmooth.com*

Red Apple Lipstick's lip glosses *redapplelipstick.com*

Una Biologicals' Vegan Peppermint Lip Balm *unabiologicals.com*

shampoo

Botanique by Himalaya Volumizing Shampoo *himalayausa.com*

Suave Professionals Almond and Shea Butter Shampoo *suave.com*

toothpaste

Crest Pro-Health Whitening Gel Toothpaste *crestprohealth.com*

Botanique by Himalaya Toothpaste *himalayausa.com*

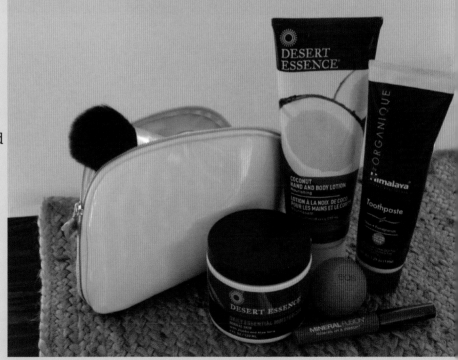

3 Ways to Use Green Tea for Glowing Skin

Chances are likely I won't be telling you anything new when I mention the benefits of green tea. That's because the brew has been timelessly touted as an antioxidant all-star as a result of its high content of flavonoids, plant-derived compounds that can pack more punch than vitamins C and E. Green tea also takes the upper hand with its bevy of catechins, disease-fighting antioxidants that are also found in red wine, chocolate, and berries. (Party time, anyone?)

The bonus? In addition to reducing risk for several cancers and other diseases, green tea also has the ability to stop oxidative damage to cells. What's that science lingo mean? Simply said, the antioxidants in green tea can help absorb some of the impact caused by free radicals, including environmental stressors like pollution, smoking, and too much sun.

That means green tea boasts a double health whammy: protecting your insides and keeping your outsides looking smashing. Take a peek at how green tea can keep you looking gorgeous with these three tips for including it in your beauty regimen.

1. Save your used bags.

Just finished a cup of green tea? Snip open the bag and empty the contents into a small bowl. Add a Tablespoon of pure honey and mix to make a paste. Dampen skin with warm water and massage the paste into skin, making small circles to ensure skin is exfoliated. Let it sit for five minutes, then rinse off. Dry skin and apply your favorite moisturizer.

2. Feeling last night's happy hour?

Take two green tea bags and run them under hot water. Allow them to cool a bit, then place them on your eyes. Lie back and enjoy the natural de-puffing sesh. Feel free to also rub the tea bags all over your face for a skin boost.

3. Make a green tea body scrub.

Brew a cup of green tea and nab about 2 Tablespoons of tea from the cup. (You can drink the rest!) Put the brewed tea in a small bowl and mix in ⅓ cup granulated sugar. You can use the scrub all over your body, including the face. Want to add a bit of moisture to your skin? Add a Tablespoon of honey to the mix and be sure to rub on rough patches, like elbows and knees.

Resource: Harvard Health Publications "Benefits of Drinking Green Tea" September 2004 (http://www.health.harvard.edu/press_releases/benefit_of_drinking_green_tea)

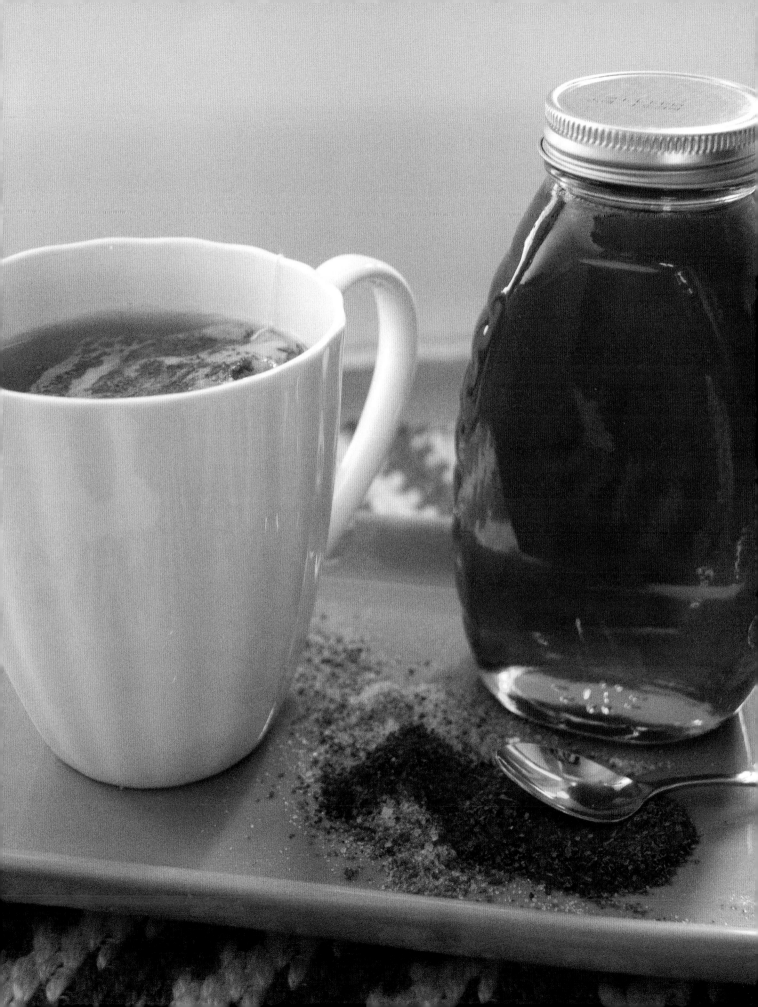

Make-at-Home Coffee Scrub
Makes about 1½ cups

It turns out that just like coffee can give your attitude a boost, it can also perk up your skin, leaving it dimple-free, toned, and absolutely glowing. This DIY scrub will reduce the appearance of cellulite and also add an extra jolt to your morning shower.

ingredients
⅓ cup coffee grounds
1 cup turbinado sugar
¼ cup olive oil
1 teaspoon vanilla extract

directions
Measure all ingredients into a medium bowl and stir until well combined. Store in a resealable container.

When ready to use, massage coffee scrub onto thigh area, rubbing in a circular motion. Rinse with warm water when finished.

NOTE: Don't have turbinado sugar? Use good ol' brown or granulated sugar instead. Same goes for olive oil—almond, baby, and grapeseed oil are all great substitutes.

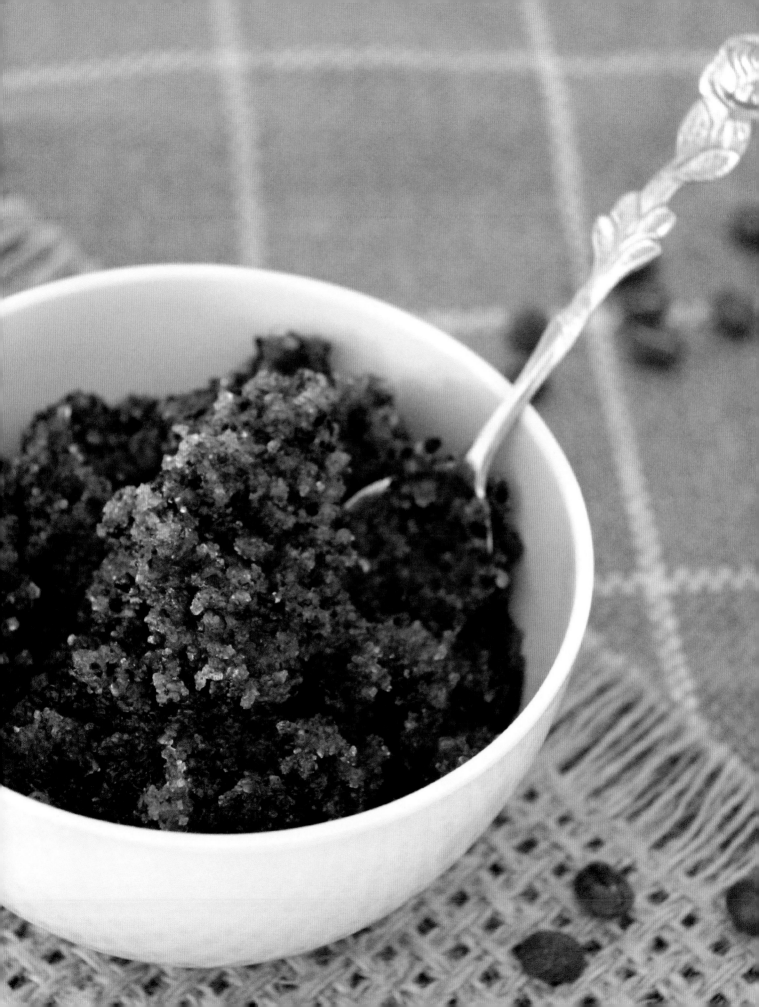

the gluten-free revolution's favorites

We all play favorites every now and then. And when it comes to food, I'll admit—I can be rather choosy. This is a list of the gluten-free products I consider to be complete rock stars. In fact, if you were to visit my house today, chances are good you would find nearly all of these products in my pantry or refrigerator. Notice that many of the companies I have listed here also offer vegan products, in addition to soy-, dairy-, and egg-free options. As always, be sure to check up on individual manufacturers every now and then to be sure they have not changed their products' ingredients.

REFRIGERATOR

Fresh Juice
- **Suja Juice:** Cold-Pressed, Organic Juices (variety of flavors, including Fiji, Purify, Fuel, Vanilla Cloud, Master Cleanse, and Glow) *sujajuice.com*
- **Organic Avenue:** Cold-Pressed, Organic Juices (variety of flavors, including Splendid Sweet Greens, Royal Red Juice, Veggie Vibe, Caring Carrot Juice, and Generous Ginger-ade Tonic) *organicavenue.com*

Supplements & Powders
- **Nutrex Hawaii:** Pure Hawaiian Spirulina Pacifica Powder *nutrex-hawaii.com*
- **Nutiva Organic:** Shelled Hempseed *nutiva.com*
- **Bob's Red Mill:** Whole Ground Flaxseed Meal *bobsredmill.com*
- **Udo's Choice:** Udo's Oil 3-6-9 Blend *oilthemachine.com*

Vegan Milk Substitutes
- **So Delicious Dairy Free:** Almond Plus™ Almond Milk Beverages (Original, Vanilla, and Unsweetened) and Coconut Milk (Original, Unsweetened Original, Vanilla, Unsweetened Vanilla and Chocolate) *sodeliciousdairyfree.com*

Vegan Cheese Substitutes
- **Daiya Cheese*:** Slices (Cheddar, Swiss, and Provolone), Wedges (Cheddar, Jack, and Jalapeño Garlic Havarti) and Shreds (Pepperjack, Mozzarella, and Cheddar)
  *Also free of dairy (casein, whey, and lactose), soy, gluten, eggs, peanuts, and tree nuts (except coconut) *daiyafoods.com*
- **Teese Vegan Cheese:** Mozzarella, Creamy Cheddar, and Cheddar
chicagoveganfoods.com

Vegan Butter Substitutes
- **Earth Balance All Natural Spreads:** Buttery Spreads (Original, Olive Oil, Soy Free, and Organic Whipped); Baking Sticks (Shortening Sticks and Vegan Buttery Sticks); and Culinary Spreads (Organic Coconut and Organic Garlic and Herbs) *earthbalancenatural.com*

Vegan Cream Cheese Substitutes
- **Daiya Cream Cheese Style Spreads*:** Plain, Chive & Onion, and Strawberry *Also free of dairy (casein, whey, and lactose), soy, gluten, eggs, peanuts, and tree nuts (except coconut) *daiyafoods.com*
- **Tofutti Better Than Cream Cheese:** Plain, Herbs & Chives, and Garlic & Herb *tofutti.com*
- **Follow Your Heart:** Vegan Gourmet Cream Cheese *followyourheart.com*

Vegan Sour Cream Substitutes
- **Tofutti:** Sour Supreme Better Than Sour Cream *tofutti.com*
- **Follow Your Heart:** Vegan Gourmet Sour Cream *followyourheart.com*

Vegan Yogurt
- **So Delicious Dairy Free:** Cultured Coconut Milk (variety of flavors, including Blueberry, Raspberry, Strawberry, Chocolate, and Vanilla) and Greek Style Cultured Coconut Milk (variety of flavors, including Blueberry, Strawberry, Raspberry, and Vanilla) *sodeliciousdairyfree.com*
- **WholeSoy & Co. Yogurt:** Wide range of flavors, including Peach, Lemon, Blueberry, Strawberry, and Vanilla

Vegan Cream Substitutes
- **So Delicious Dairy Free Coconut Milk "Creamers":** Original, Vanilla, and Hazelnut *sodeliciousdairyfree.com*

Vegan Mayonnaise Substitute

- **Follow Your Heart:** Vegenaise (Original, Reduced Fat, and Grapeseed Oil *followyourheart.com*

Salad Dressings

- **Annie's:** Dressings (variety of flavors, including Lite Honey Mustard, Lite Raspberry Vinaigrette, Tuscany Italian, and Fat Free Mango Vinaigrette)
  Note: Not all Annie's dressings are gluten-free, so be sure to check labels! *annies.com*
- **Newman's Own:** Dressings (variety of flavors, including Balsamic Vinaigrette, Lite Honey Mustard, Lite Lime Vinaigrette, and Poppy Seed Dressing)
  Note: Not all Newman's Own dressings are gluten-free, so be sure to check labels! *newmansown.com*

Other Condiments

- **Annie's:** Organic Honey Mustard and Organic Sweet & Spicy BBQ Sauce
  Note: Not all Annie's condiments are gluten-free, so be sure to check labels! *annies.com*
- **Thai Kitchen:** Red Curry and Roasted Red Chili pastes; Peanut Satay Sauce; and Red, Yellow, and Green Curry 10-Minute Simmer Sauces *thaikitchen.com*
- **Eden:** Mirin Rice Cooking Wine *edenfoods.com*
- **San-J:** Gluten-Free Tamari (regular and reduced sodium) and Gluten-Free Asian Cooking Sauces (variety of flavors, including Teriyaki, Sweet & Tangy, and Thai Peanut) *san-j.com*

Beer and Cider

- **Green's:** Belgian Ales (Quest Tripel Ale, Endeavour Dubbel Ale, and Discovery Amber Ale) *glutenfreebeers.co.uk*
- **Angry Orchard:** Hard Cider (Crisp Apple, Traditional Dry, Apple Ginger, and Elderflower) *angryorchard.com*
- **New Planet:** Pale, Amber, Raspberry, and Blonde ales *newplanetbeer.com*

FREEZER

Veggie Burgers

- **Sunshine Burgers:** Variety of flavors, including Original, Barbecue, Falafel, and Garden Herb *sunshineburger.com*
- **Hilary's Eat Well:** Hemp & Greens, Adzuki Bean Burger, and Veggie Burger *hilaryseatwell.com*

Burritos

- **Amy's Kitchen:** Gluten-Free Burritos (Cheddar, Indian Aloo Mattar, Teriyaki, Tofu Breakfast Scramble, and Non-Dairy)
  Note: Not all Amy's burritos are gluten-free, so be sure to check labels! *amys.com*

Pasta & Grains

- **Conte's Pasta:** Raviolis (Cheese and Spinach & Cheese) and Pierogies
  Note: Not all Conte's products are gluten-free, so be sure to check labels! *contespasta.com*
- **365 Everyday Value Organic Quinoa:** White Quinoa and Quinoa With Vegetables *wholefoodsmarket.com*

Pizza

- **Daiya Pizzas*:** Cheeze Lover's, Fire-Roasted Vegetable, Mushroom & Roasted Garlic and Margherita
  *Also free of dairy (casein, whey and lactose), soy, gluten, eggs, peanuts, and tree nuts (except coconut) *daiyafoods.com*

Bread, Bagels & Tortillas

- **Against the Grain Gourmet:** Baguettes (Original and Rosemary); Rolls (Rosemary and Pumpernickel); Bagels (Sesame and Sun-Dried Tomato & Basil); and Pizza Shells *againstthegraingourmet.com*

- **Three Bakers:** Whole Grain Rye Style and 7 Ancient Grains breads *threebakers.com*
- **Rudi's Gluten-Free Bakery:** Tortillas & Wraps (Plain, Fiesta, and Spinach) and Multigrain Hamburger Buns
  Note: Not all Rudi's bakery products are gluten-free, so be sure to check labels! *rudisbakery.com*

Waffles
- **Van's Natural Foods:** Gluten-Free Waffles (variety of flavors, including Blueberry, Apple Cinnamon, Totally Natural, and Ancient Grains Original)
  Note: Not all Van's products are gluten-free, so be sure to check labels! *vansfoods.com*
- **Nature's Path:** Gluten-Free Waffles (Homestyle and Buckwheat Wildberry)
  Note: Not all Nature's Path products are gluten-free, so be sure to check labels! *naturespath.com*

Frozen Desserts
- **Jeni's Splendid Ice Creams:** Signature Flavors (variety of flavors, including Brown Butter Almond Brittle Ice Cream, Black Coffee, Dark Chocolate, Pistachio and Honey, The Buckeye State, and Salty Caramel) and Macaroon Sandwiches (Chocolate Hazelnut, Mango Pistachio, Orchid Vanilla, and Salty Caramel with Smoked Almonds)
  Note: Not all Jeni's products are gluten-free, so be sure to check labels! *jenis.com*
- **Edy's/Dreyer's Ice Creams:** Slow Churned (variety of flavors, including Peanut Butter Cup, French Vanilla, and Mint Chocolate Chip) and Grand (variety of flavors, including Espresso Chip, Chocolate Peanut Butter Cup, and Mocha Almond Fudge) *edys.com*

Vegan Frozen Desserts
- **So Delicious Dairy Free:** Coconut Milk Frozen Desserts (variety of flavors, including Cookie Dough, Chocolate Peanut Butter Swirl, Green Tea, and

Turtle Trails); Almond Milk Frozen Desserts (variety of flavors, including Mocha Almond Fudge, Mint Chip and Chocolate); and Purely Decadent Pints (variety of flavors, including Peanut Butter Zig Zag, Chocolate Obsession, and Pomegranate Chip)

Note: Not all So Delicious frozen desserts are gluten-free, so be sure to check labels! *sodeliciousdairyfree.com*

PANTRY

Vitamins & Powders

- **Vega Sport:** Performance Protein Powder (Chocolate, Vanilla, and Berry) *vegasport.com*
- **Nutiva Organic:** Organic Hemp Protein and Organic Chia Seed *nutiva.com*
- **Navitas Naturals:** Raw Cacao Powder and Raw Maca Powder *navitasnaturals.com*

Pasta

- **Ancient Harvest:** Elbows, Linguine, Spaghetti, Rotelle, Shells, and Garden Pagodas *quinoa.net*
- **Schar:** Multigrain Penne Rigate, Tagliatelle, Anellini, and Spaghetti *schar.com*
- **BiAglut*:** Variety of pasta, including Fusilli, Penne, Ditalini, and Shells *Also wheat-, milk-, and egg-free *biaglutusa.com*
- **Jovial Foods:** Brown Rice Pasta (Spaghetti, Penne, and Fusilli)
  Note: Not all Jovial Foods products are gluten-free, so be sure to check labels! *jovialfoods.com*
- **Tinkyada:** Brown Rice Lasagna Noodles *tinkyada.com*

Cereals & Oats

- **Purely Elizabeth Ancient Grain Granola Cereal:** Original, Pumpkin Fig, Blueberry Hemp, and Cranberry Pecan *purelyelizabeth.com*

- **Nature's Path:** Envirokidz Cereals (Peanut Butter Pandas, Leapin' Lemurs and Gorilla Munch); Qi'a Chia, Buckwheat & Hemp Cereals (Original, Apple Cinnamon, and Cranberry Vanilla); and Nature's Path Mesa Sunrise Flakes with Raisins
  Note: Not all Nature's Path products are gluten-free, so be sure to check labels! *naturespath.com*
- **KIND Healthy Snacks Granola:** Peanut Butter, Blueberry Clusters with Flax Seeds, Cinnamon Oat Clusters with Flax Seeds, and Oats & Honey Clusters with Toasted Coconut *kindsnacks.com*
- **Bob's Red Mill Gluten-Free Oats:** Steel Cut and Whole Grain Rolled Oats
  Note: Not all Bob's Red Mill products are gluten-free, so be sure to check labels! *bobsredmill.com*
- **Cocomama Foods Heat-and-Eat Quinoa Cereals:** Banana Cinnamon, Honey Almond, and Orange Cranberry *cocomamafoods.com*

Pizza Crust
- **Schar:** Gluten-Free Pizza Base *schar.com*
- **Bob's Red Mill:** Whole Grain Gluten-Free Pizza Crust Mix
  Note: Not all Bob's Red Mill products are gluten-free, so be sure to check labels! *bobsredmill.com*

Food Bars
- **KIND Healthy Snacks*:** Variety of flavors, including Peanut Butter Dark Chocolate + Protein, Almond & Coconut, Peanut Butter & Strawberry, Pomegranate Blueberry Pistachio + Antioxidants, Dark Chocolate Cinnamon Pecan, and Dark Chocolate Nuts & Sea Salt
  *Offers many vegan options kindsnacks.com
- **LARABARS*:** Variety of flavors, including Apple Pie, Banana Bread, Blueberry Muffin, Peanut Butter Cookie, Pecan Pie, and Chocolate Chip Cookie Dough
  *Offers many vegan and soy-free options larabar.com

Crackers

- **Crunchmaster Multi-Seed Crackers:** Original, Sea salt, White Cheddar, Toasted Onion, Roasted Garlic, and Rosemary & Olive Oil *crunchmaster.com*
- **Mary's Gone Crackers:** Crackers (Original, Herb, and Onion) and Pretzel Sticks (Sea Salt and Curry) *marysgonecrackers.com*
- **Sesmark:** Savory Rice Thins (Original, Teriyaki, and Toasted Onion) and Garlic and Rice Thins (Sesame and Brown Rice)
  Note: Not all Sesmark products are gluten-free, so be sure to check labels! *sesmark.com*

Prepared Mixes

- **Pamela's:** Cornbread and Muffin Mix *pamelasproducts.com*
- **Betty Crocker:** Gluten-Free Bisquick Waffle Mix, Chocolate Brownie Mix, and Sugar Cookie Mix *bettycrocker.com*
- **1-2-3 Gluten-Free Baking Mixes:** Divinely Decadent Brownies *123glutenfree.com*
- **Chebe:** Pizza Crust, Foccaccia, and All-Purpose Bread mixes *chebe.com*

Flour

- **Bob's Red Mill Gluten-Free Flours:** Variety of options, including almond meal, tapioca flour, cornstarch, coconut flour, brown rice flour, arrowroot starch, white rice flour, and xanthan gum
  Note: Not all Bob's Red Mill products are gluten-free, so be sure to check labels! *bobsredmill.com*
- **Outrageous Baking:** All-Purpose Baking Flour Mix *outrageousbaking.com*

Baking Sugars, Coconut & Chocolate Chips

- **Shiloh Farms:** Coconut Sugar *shilohfarms.com*
- **Lundberg Family Farms:** Organic Sweet Dreams Brown Rice Syrup *lundberg.com*
- **Let's Do®...Organic:** Unsweetened Shredded Coconut *edwardandsons.com*
- **Enjoy Life Foods*:** Mini Chips and Mega Chunks
  *Also dairy-, nut-, and soy-free *enjoylifefoods.com*

Grains
- **Ancient Harvest:** Quinoa (Traditional and Inca Red) and Quinoa Flakes *quinoa.net*
- **Lundberg Family Farms:** Rice (variety of rice and rice mixes, including Short Grain, Basmati Brown, Arborio, and Jasmine Brown rices); Risotto (variety of flavors, including Alfredo, Porcini Mushroom, Butternut Squash, and Italian Herb); and Brown Rice Couscous (Plain Original, Savory Herb, and Roasted Garlic & Olive Oil) *lundberg.com*

Pasta Sauce & Pesto
- **Mezzeta:** Red Sauces (variety of flavors, including Roasted Garlic, Tomato Basil, Creamy Vodka Style Marinara, and Porcini Mushroom) and Homemade Style Basil Pesto *mezzetta.com*
- **Classico:** Red Sauces (variety of flavors, including Caramelized Onion and Roasted Garlic, Fire-Roasted Tomato and Garlic, Mushroom and Ripe Olives and Portobello, Crimini & Champignon Mushroom) *classico.com*

Other Condiments
- **Maya Kaimal Indian Simmer Sauces:** Tikka Masala, Kashmiri Curry Butter Masala, and Madras Curry *mayakaimal.com*

index

A
almonds, 15, 28, 49, 97, 154
almond milk, 207
apple
   Apple Cheesecake Pie, 148
   Beet-iful Ginger Apple Smoothie, 36
appetizer
   Asian Lettuce Wraps, 88
   Black Bean & Banana Salsa, 81
   Curried Chickpea Bites, 75
   Ginger Sesame Seed Cucumbers, 79
   Open-Faced Polenta Caprese
   Sandwiches, 72
   Snails & Seeds Dinner Rolls, 83
   Stuffed Mini Red Potatoes, 87
   Sweet Potato French Fry Dip, 76
applesauce, 14
asparagus
   Goat Cheese & Asparagus Quiche
    Cups, 51
   Grapefruit & Asparagus Salad, 98
avocado, 15, 35, 136, 147

B
bananas
   Black Bean & Banana Salsa, 81
   Frozen Chocolate Banana Peanut
    Bites, 142
   Peanut Butter & Banana Cupcakes, 158
Banana Bread Quinoa Cereal, 47
bars
   Raw Sour Cherry Almond
    Bars, 49
   store bought, 213
barre
   5 Ballet-Inspired Exercises for a
    Perky Booty, 191

beans
   Black Bean & Banana Salsa, 81
   Black-Eyed Pea Quinoa Salad, 100
   No-Fuss Burrito in a Bowl, 136
   Weeklong Chili, 133
beauty
   Green Tea for Glowing Skin, 202
   gluten-free products, 201
   Make-At-Home Coffee Scrub, 204
beer, 209
beet
   Beet-iful Ginger Apple Smoothie, 36
   Purifying Beet & Cabbage Salad, 97
beta-carotene, 76, 97
blenders, 19, 29
blog
   The G-Spot Revolution, 2
bread
   Snails & Seeds Dinner Rolls, 83
   store bought, 17, 210-11, 214
breakfast
   Banana Bread Quinoa Cereal, 47
   Goat Cheese & Asparagus
    Quiche Cups, 51
   Mushroom Potato Crust Quiche, 57
   Orange Fig Pecan Granola, 40
   Peanut Butter Coconut Quinoa
    Granola, 45
   Raspberry Lemonade Doughnuts, 58
   Raw Sour Cherry Almond Bars, 49
   Sweet Potato Spinach Quiche, 54
   Tropical Pineapple Yogurt, 43
brownies, 214
Brussels sprouts, 15, 28
Brown Butter & Thyme Pasta, 108
Build-Your-Own Smoothie, 28
butter substitute, 208

C

cabbage
  Purifying Beet & Cabbage Salad, 97
cardiovascular health
  Cardio Pilates, 185
  On Running, 179
carrot
  Brown Sugar Glazed Carrots &
    Parsnips, 95
  Orange Carrot Ginger Sunrise
    Smoothie, 26
cauliflower
  Cauliflower Rice, 123
  Veggie Stuffed Peppers, 124
celiac disease, 2, 6
cereal
  Banana Bread Quinoa Cereal, 47
cereal & oats, 212–13
cheese
  Cheesy Tuna Tater Pie, 112–11
  Goat Cheese & Asparagus Quiche
    Cups, 51
  Pineapple Goat Cheese Pizza, 118
cheese substitute
cheesecake
  Apple Cheesecake Pie, 148
cherry
  Raw Sour Cherry Almond Bars, 49
chickpea
  Curried Chickpea Bites, 75
  Honey Dijon Chickpea &
    Olive Pizza, 120
children
chili
  Weeklong Chili, 133
chocolate
  Chocolate Mint Dessert Smoothie, 147
  Frozen Chocolate Banana Peanut
    Bites, 142
  Nuts-About-Chocolate Clusters, 154

cider, 209
coconut
  Peanut Butter Coconut Quinoa
    Granola, 45
coconut oil, 17, 43
coffee
  Make-At-Home Coffee Scrub, 204
  Raspberry Coffee Pick-Me-Up, 30
condiments, 209, 215
cookies
  Classic Oatmeal Raisin Cookies, 152
  Pistachio Crusted Orange Cookies, 140
  Sunflower Butter & Jelly Cookies, 156
cookware, 20–1
crackers, store-bought, 214
cream substitute, 208
cream cheese substitute, 20
cucumber
  Cucumber Lime Water, 32
  Ginger Sesame Seed Cucumbers, 79
cupcake
  Peanut Butter & Banana Cupcakes, 158
curry
  Curried Chickpea Bites, 75

D

dairy-free milk, 16, 207
dessert
  Apple Cheesecake Pie, 148
  Chocolate Mint Dessert Smoothie, 147
  Classic Oatmeal Raisin Cookies, 152
  Frozen Chocolate Banana Peanut
    Bites, 142
  Nuts-About-Chocolate Clusters, 154
  Oatmeal Crust, 145
  Peanut Butter & Banana Cupcakes, 158
  Peanut Butter Protein Fudge, 151
  Pistachio Crusted Orange Cookies, 140
  Sunflower Butter & Jelly Cookies, 156

doughnuts
    Raspberry Lemonade Doughnuts, 58
dressings, salad
    Honey Mustard Dressing, 62
    Lemon Garlic Cleansing Dressing, 65
    Traditional Balsamic Dressing, 64

E
Edible Flowers and Orange Water, 32
eggs
    Goat Cheese & Asparagus Quiche
      Cups, 51
    Mushroom Potato Crust Quiche, 57
    Sweet Potato Spinach Quiche, 54
eggplant
    Sloppy Faux Joes, 130
entrée
    Brown Butter & Thyme Pasta, 108
    Cauliflower Rice, 123
    Cheesy Tuna Tater Pie, 112–13
    Fiesta Quinoa Stir-fry, 110
    Honey Dijon Chickpea & Olive
      Pizza, 120
    Mushroom Stroganoff, 134
    No-Fuss Burrito in a Bowl, 136
    Parchment Paper Steamed Salmon, 107
    Pimp Yo' Potato, 126
    Pineapple Goat Cheese Pizza, 118
    Pineapple Sesame Tofu, 128
    Raw Zucchini Pasta, 115
    Raw Zucchini Pesto Noodles, 117
    Sloppy Faux Joes, 130
    Spaghetti Squash Pasta, 104
    Veggie Stuffed Peppers, 124
    Weeklong Chili, 133

F
family
    Snails & Seeds Dinner Rolls, 83

fats and oils, 14, 28
fennel, 107
fitness
    4 Yoga Poses for Reducing Head Pain,
      169
    5 Ballet-Inspired Exercises for a Perky
      Booty, 191
    Cardio Pilates, 185
    Drool-Worthy Sleepy Time Yoga
      Sequence, 173
    On Running, 179
    Take-'Em-Anywhere Yoga Poses, 163
fish
    Cheesy Tuna Tater Pie, 112–113
    Parchment Paper Steamed Salmon, 107
flaxseed egg, 58, 75, 140, 152, 156, 158, 207
flaxseed meal, 16, 28, 40, 45
flour
    Gluten-Free All-Purpose Baking
      Mix, 144
    store bought, 14, 214
food processor, 19
freezer items, 17, 210-212
frozen desserts, 211–12
fruit, 16
fudge
    Peanut Butter Protein Fudge, 151

G
garlic
    Lemon Garlic Cleansing Dressing, 65
ginger
    Beet-iful Ginger Apple Smoothie, 36
    Orange Carrot Ginger Sunrise
      Smoothie, 26
Gluten-Free Beauty Products, 21, 201
Grapefruit & Asparagus Salad, 98
grains, 14, 210
granola
    Orange Fig Pecan Granola, 40

Peanut Butter Coconut Quinoa
    Granola, 45
greens, 15–6, 28, 63
Green Machine Smoothie, 24

H
headaches
    4 Yoga Poses for Reducing Head
        Pain, 169
healthy juices
honey
    Honey Dijon Chickpea & Olive
        Pizza, 120
    Honey Mustard Dressing, 62
hummus, 17

I
ice cream, 211–212
immune system, 26, 35, 36, 76
infused water, 32–33
iron, 24, 36, 63

J
juicers, 29
juice, 207
Juicing vs. Blending, 29

K
kale, 28
kiwi
    Hair & Skin Kiwi Booster, 35
knives, 20

L
lemon
    Lemon Garlic Cleansing Dressing, 65
    Raspberry Lemonade Doughnuts, 58
lettuce varieties, 63

M
maple syrup, 14
marinade
    Sesame Marinade, 66
migraine
    4 Yoga Poses for Reducing Head
        Pain, 169
mint
    Chocolate Mint Dessert Smoothie, 147
    Strawberry Maca Mint Smoothie, 25
mixer, 19
mixes, store bought, 214
mushroom
    Mushroom Potato Crust Quiche, 57
    Mushroom Stroganoff, 134
    Sloppy Faux Joes, 130
mustard
    Honey Mustard Dressing, 62
    Traditional Balsamic Dressing, 64

N
nutmeg, 14, 51
nuts
    Frozen Chocolate Banana Peanut
        Bites, 142
    Nuts-About-Chocolate Clusters, 154
    Orange Fig Pecan Granola, 40
    Roasted Walnut Herb Pesto, 68

O
oats & cereal, 212–13
oatmeal
    Classic Oatmeal Raisin Cookies, 152
    Oatmeal Crust, 145
olive
    Honey Dijon Chickpea & Olive Pizza, 120
oils, 14
onions, 15, 53
orange

Orange Carrot Ginger Sunrise
      Smoothie, 26
Orange Fig Pecan Granola, 40
Pistachio Crusted Orange Cookies, 140

P
pantry, 13-15, 212–215
parsley, 15
parsnips
      Brown Sugar Glazed Carrots &
            Parsnips, 95
pasta
      Brown Butter & Thyme Pasta, 108
      Mushroom Stroganoff, 134
      store bought, 210, 212
pasta sauce & pesto, store bought, 215
peanut butter
      Peanut Butter & Banana Cupcakes, 158
      Peanut Butter Coconut Quinoa
            Granola, 45
      Peanut Butter Protein Fudge, 151
pecan
      Orange Fig Pecan Granola, 40
pepper, bell
      Fiesta Quinoa Stir-fry, 110
      Sloppy Faux Joes, 130
      Veggie Stuffed Peppers, 124
pesto
      Raw Zucchini Pesto Noodles, 117
      Roasted Walnut Herb Pesto, 68
pesto, store bought, 215
pie
      Apple Cheesecake Pie, 148
      Oatmeal Crust, 145
pilates
      Cardio Pilates, 185
pineapple
      Pineapple Goat Cheese Pizza, 118
      Pineapple Sesame Tofu, 128

Tropical Pineapple Yogurt, 43
Pistachio Crusted Orange Cookies, 140
pizza
      Honey Dijon Chickpea & Olive
            Pizza, 120
      Pineapple Goat Cheese Pizza, 118
      frozen, 210
pizza crust, store bought, 210, 213–14
polenta
      Open-Faced Polenta Caprese
            Sandwiches, 72
Post-Workout Smoothie, 34
potassium, 34
potato
      Mushroom Potato Crust Quiche, 57
      Pimp Yo' Potato, 126
      Stuffed Mini Red Potatoes, 87
      Sweet Potato French Fry Dip, 76
      Sweet Potato Spinach Quiche, 54
protein powder
      Peanut Butter Protein Fudge, 151
pumpkin, 14

Q
quiche
      Goat Cheese & Asparagus Quiche
            Cups, 51
      Mushroom Potato Crust Quiche, 57
      Sweet Potato Spinach Quiche, 54
quinoa
      Banana Bread Quinoa Cereal, 47
      Black-Eyed Pea Quinoa Salad, 100
      Fiesta Quinoa Stir-fry, 110
      Peanut Butter Coconut Quinoa
            Granola, 45
      Rainbow Quinoa Salad, 92

R
raw
      Raw Sour Cherry Almond Bars, 49

Raw Zucchini Pasta, 115
Raw Zucchini Pesto Noodles, 117
raspberry
    Raspberry Coffee Pick-Me-Up
        Smoothie, 30
    Raspberry Lemonade Doughnuts, 58
    Raspberries and Mint Water, 32
refrigerator items, 15–17, 207–209
rice, 14, 215
rosemary, 13
running
    On Running, 179

S
salad
    Black-Eyed Pea Quinoa Salad, 100
    Grapefruit & Asparagus Salad, 98
    Purifying Beet & Cabbage Salad, 97
    Rainbow Quinoa Salad, 92
salad dressing
    Traditional Balsamic Dressing, 64
    Honey Mustard Dressing, 62
    Lemon Garlic Cleansing Dressing, 65
salad dressings, pre-made, 17, 209
salsa
    Black Bean & Banana Salsa, 81
sage, 17
sandwich
    Open-Faced Polenta Caprese
        Sandwiches, 72
    Sloppy Faux Joes, 130
scrub
    green tea body scrub, 202
    Make-At-Home Coffee Scrub, 204
sesame
    Ginger Sesame Seed Cucumbers, 79
    Pineapple Sesame Tofu, 128
    Sesame Marinade, 66
    Snails & Seeds Dinner Rolls, 83
simmer sauce, store bought, 215
skin health
    Green Tea for Glowing Skin, 202

sleep
    Drool-Worthy Sleepy Time Yoga
        Sequence, 173
smoothies
    Beet-iful Ginger Apple Smoothie, 36
    Build-Your-Own Smoothie, 28
    Chocolate Mint Dessert Smoothie, 147
    Green Machine Smoothie, 24
    Hair & Skin Kiwi Booster, 35
    Orange Carrot Ginger Sunrise
        Smoothie, 26
    Post-Workout Smoothie, 34
    Raspberry Coffee Pick-Me-Up, 30
    Strawberry Maca Mint Smoothie, 25
sour cream substitute, 208
soy sauce, gluten-free, 14, 209
spinach
    Sweet Potato Spinach Quiche, 54
spirulina, 16, 28, 207
squash
    Spaghetti Squash Pasta, 104
strawberries
    Strawberry Maca Mint Smoothie, 25
sugar
    coconut sugar, 14, 140, 214
sunflower
    Sunflower Butter & Jelly Cookies, 156
Supplements & Powders, 21, 207
Sweet and Sour Caponata, 69
sweet potato
    Sweet Potato French Fry Dip, 76
    Sweet Potato Spinach Quiche, 54

T
tamari, 14, 209
tea
    Green Tea for Glowing Skin, 202
thyme, 14, 17, 108
Tropical Pineapple Yogurt, 43
    Brown Butter & Thyme Pasta, 108
tofu
    Pineapple Sesame Tofu, 128
tomato

Open-Faced Polenta Caprese
    Sandwiches, 72

V
vegan
    Apple Cheesecake Pie, 148
        Crust
    Black Bean & Banana Salsa, 81
    Brown Butter & Thyme Pasta, 108
    Chocolate Mint Dessert Smoothie, 147
    Classic Oatmeal Raisin Cookies, 152
    Curried Chickpea Bites, 75
    dairy substitutes
        butter, 208
        cheese, 207
        cream, 208
        cream cheese, 208
        milk, 207
        mayonnaise, 209
        sour cream, 208
        yogurt, 208
    Fiesta Quinoa Stir-fry, 110
    Frozen Banana Peanut Bites, 142
    frozen desserts, 211–12
    Ginger Sesame Seed Cucumbers, 79
    Honey Dijon Chickpea & Olive Pizza, 12
    Mushroom Stroganoff, 134
    No-Fuss Burrito in a Bowl, 136
    Nuts-About-Chocolate Clusters, 154
    Oatmeal Crust, 145
    Peanut Butter & Banana Cupcakes, 158
    Peanut Butter Protein Fudge, 151
    Pimp Yo' Potato, 126
    Pineapple Goat Cheese Pizza, 118
    Pineapple Sesame Tofu, 128
    Pistachio Crusted Orange Cookies, 140
    Raw Zucchini Pesto Noodles, 117

Sloppy Faux Joes, 130
    Stuffed Mini Red Potatoes, 87
    Sunflower Butter & Jelly Cookies, 156
    Sweet Potato French Fry Dip, 76
Veggie Stuffed Peppers, 124
    Weeklong Veggie Chili, 133
vegetables, 15–17
vitamins & powders, 212

W
waffles, store-bought, 211
walk-run, 181
walnut
    Roasted Walnut Herb Pesto, 68

Y
yoga
    4 Yoga Poses for Reducing Head
        Pain, 169
    Drool-Worthy Sleepy Time Yoga
        Sequence, 173
    Take-'Em-Anywhere Yoga Poses, 163
yogurt
    Tropical Pineapple Yogurt, 43
    vegan, 208

Z
zucchini
    Raw Zucchini Pasta, 115
    Raw Zucchini Pesto Noodles, 117

Acknowledgments

First and foremost, thank you from the bottom of my heart to my readers. You are the icing on my gluten-free cupcake and I am grateful for you each day.

To my parents, Mary and Dave Shannon, for believing in me every single moment of this blessed life I am leading. You've supported every dream and every crazy aspiration—I truly could not have done it without you. I love you up to the sky and back down again.

To Amanda, Luke, and Isaac, you are my siblings by the grace of this universe, but you are my best friends because we choose to be.

To Dan, my husband, you are more than I ever could have asked for in a friend and life partner. Thank you for being my cheerleader, sounding board, second photographer, and on many late nights—sanity. I adore you.

To my grandmother, Caroline Shorkey, for teaching me to always believe in magic. I still do and always will.

To my extended family—aunts, uncles, cousins, brother-in-law, the Karasiks, the Bloemers and friends—for all of the love and support.

To my editor, Brandon Schultz, for never faltering in his belief that this message is one that should be shared with everyone. I wouldn't be here without your confidence in me and this book.

To my kitties, Cooper, Emerson, Madeline, and Simon. Sometimes, you're the only "people" I need for the day. And for taking turns as my lap cat throughout this writing process!

To LA Finfinger, Anna Gilbert Zupon, Maggie Ryan, and Misty Lynne Cauthen for sharing their individual passions for fitness. I am so thankful for each one of you.

To South Hills Power Yoga and Stray Dog Yoga studios in Pittsburgh. Your beautiful spaces made much of this fitness section a possibility.

And, finally, to each one of the health and wellness gurus who inspire me. You have paved the way since the very first moment I opened one of your books and continue to do so to this very day.

Oven Temperatures

Fahrenheit	Celcius	Gas Mark
225°	110°	¼
250°	120°	½
275°	140°	1
300°	150°	2
325°	160°	3
350°	180°	4
375°	190°	5
400°	200°	6
425°	220°	7
450°	230°	8

Metric and Imperial Conversions

(These conversions are rounded for convenience)

Ingredient	Cups/Tablespoons/ Teaspoons	Ounces	Grams/Milliliters
Butter	1 cup=16 table-spoons= 2 sticks	8 ounces	230 grams
Cream cheese	1 Tablespoon	0.5 ounce	14.5 grams
Cheese, shredded	1 cup	4 ounces	110 grams
Cornstarch	1 Tablespoon	0.3 ounce	8 grams
Fruit, dried	1 cup	4 ounces	120 grams
Fruits or veggies, chopped	1 cup	5 to 7 ounces	145 to 200 grams
Fruits or veggies, pureed	1 cup	8.5 ounces	245 grams
Gluten-free Flour	1 cup/1 Tablespoon	4.5 ounces/0.3 ounce	125 grams/8 grams
Honey, maple syrup, or corn syrup	1 Tablespoon	.75 ounce	20 grams
Liquids: cream, milk, water, or juice	1 cup	8 fluid ounces	240 milliliters
Oats	1 cup	5.5 ounces	150 grams
Salt	1 teaspoon	0.2 ounces	6 grams
Spices: cinna-mon, cloves, ginger, or nutmeg (ground)	1 teaspoon	0.2 ounce	5 milliliters
Sugar, brown, firmly packed	1 cup	7 ounces	200 grams
Sugar, white	1 cup/1 Tablespoon	7 ounces/0.5 ounce	200 grams/12.5 grams
Vanilla extract	1 teaspoon	0.2 ounce	4 grams

Lifestyle Goals

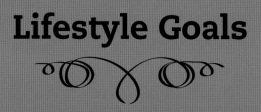

Recipe Notes